Hospital Administration For Veterinary Staff

Thomas H. Pettit, DVM
Farnsworth Hall
State University of New York
Delhi, NY 13753

Technical Editor: Joann Colville, DVM
Book Editor: Paul W. Pratt, VMD
Associate Editor: Elizabeth V. Hillyer, VMD
Production Manager: Elisabeth S. Stein
Production Assistant: Matthew B. Davidson

American Veterinary Publications, Inc.
5782 Thornwood Drive
Goleta, CA 93117

Library of Congress Catalog Card Number: 93-74972

ISBN 0-939674-53-X

Printed and Bound in the United States of America

Preface

An increasing number of veterinary hospitals are using the services of a hospital manager. Currently, most managers are either veterinarians with an interest and success in management, or are business-educated professionals; few are technicians or lay staff. More hospital staff members will become hospital managers as their experience in practice increases and their interest in management peaks. This is a natural development for staff members; however, additional college business courses may be required to supplement the hands-on practice experience.

Hospital staff members are expected to be proficient in client relations, scheduling, client education, records and telephone answering. Eventually, they will need to understand computers, inventory control and drug ordering. Employee supervision is another task that a staff member may be required to do.

This text is an attempt to draw these many facets of hospital management between 2 covers. It is designed for the student, giving basic information about management. In addition, graduate technicians and lay personnel may find the book a handy reference as they develop more sophisticated management tools. Veterinarians may wish to have the book in their library to loan to employees.

The book is dedicated to the many veterinary technicians and veterinary technician educators, past and present, who have contributed so much to this profession.

Thomas H. Pettit, DVM

This page intentionally left blank.

Contents

This page intentionally left blank.

1

Standard Operating Procedures

Successful veterinary practices are built on a solid foundation of good personnel. The mortar binding the hospital and personnel together is a *standard operating procedure* (SOP). Some of these policies are given to hospital staff members in written form; others may be verbally communicated. Unfortunately, some policy statements are only implied; however, you are expected to implement many of them when dealing with clients. The advantage of a written policy is obvious, and attempts should be made in veterinary hospital management to have operating procedures standardized, written, understood and available for all the staff.

The SOP should include hospital policies on preventive medicine, including vaccinations, parasite control and neutering. Proper nutrition and dental, ear and eye care are also part of preventive medicine. The SOP may also include hospital policy on presurgical preparation and postoperative care for its patients. Each practice will have slightly different policies. Some general principles are described here.

Patient Health Folders For Clients

Veterinary hospitals may provide the animal owner with individualized health record folders. These folders vary in size and content but all hold general information for the client about his or her pet. They are not maintained in the same detail as hospital medical records, but are used to document illness conditions and vaccination status. Some clients are very conscientious in completing the folders; others never use them.

You should explain the value of health folders and encourage their use. Be sure that pertinent data are recorded, and add copies of vaccination certificates and other documents at each visit. Positive reinforcement will encourage clients to participate. These folders are good for client relations.

Vaccinations

Vaccinations are administered to stimulate immunity against certain diseases. Young animals are typically given a series of vaccinations, following which "booster" vaccinations are given on a regular basis, usually once a year.

The schedule of administration may vary for the different types of vaccinations. Moreover, the route of vaccine administration is important. For example, some rabies vaccines must be given by the intramuscular route, while some feline herpesvirus and calicivirus vaccines are administered intranasally. There may be limitations on vaccine use; many vaccines cannot be given to pregnant animals or when animals are ill. Be familiar with package inserts and follow the manufacturers' recommendations and the hospital vaccination protocol. The veterinarian will make final decisions regarding vaccine administration.

Each animal species requires a different set of vaccinations. A vaccine should never be administered to a species other than that for which it is intended both for legal reasons and because it could cause an unforeseen reaction, resulting in a serious problem. The vaccination protocol for dogs and cats is relatively standard across the United States, whereas the vaccination protocol for horses, cattle, swine and small ruminants varies according to geographic area and use of the animal. Moreover, state and federal laws require certain vaccinations for animals that are to be transported, and show and fair regulations may dictate that certain vaccines are necessary for entry onto the grounds. Hospital staff members should keep current copies of local regulations.

The client's first visit with their pet is a good time for the veterinary technician to discuss infectious diseases and the importance of preventive health through vaccination. Describe each disease for which a vaccination is planned. Clients will be more likely to adhere to the recommended vaccination schedules if they are aware of which diseases can be avoided by vaccination. Take this time to review the hospital's vaccination reminder system and recommendations for neutering. Solicit any questions from the client.

Always advise the client of potential side effects from vaccination. These include soreness and swelling at the injection site and possibly a slight fever or temporary lameness. Because these problems should be transitory, caution the owner to report any prolonged problems.

Parasite Control

Dogs and Cats

Dogs and cats are screened for intestinal parasites by performing routine fecal examinations. Treatment is administered according to test results. Alternatively, some veterinarians may prefer routine deworming of certain animals, such as puppies and kittens or those that frequent a particular park. External parasitism is diagnosed during an office visit by physical examination, sometimes with microscopic examination of skin scrapings. Signs of external parasitism can include head shaking, hair loss and excessive scratching.

Staff members are often required to speak with clients about parasite control. Client education should include a description of possible parasites and their enzootic potential, and a discussion of the importance of treatment, future surveillance and environmental control of the parasite.

Heartworm Disease

Canine heartworm disease is prevalent in many parts of the country. Prevention of the disease is much safer and less costly than treatment. The recommended preventive program varies according to geographic area and the specific medication used by the hospital. Routine screening is generally recommended and, again, the protocol for this varies slightly from hospital to hospital.

Client education about heartworm disease is essential to motivate clients to adhere to the preventive program. The veterinary technician should be well-versed in the life cycle, clinical signs, diagnosis and prevention of heartworm disease.

Horses, Ruminants, Swine

Control of intestinal parasites in horses, ruminants and swine usually comprises routine scheduled dewormings, pasture management and sanitation of enclosures. Fecal examinations can be performed, if necessary, to confirm a diagnosis of intestinal parasitism. Milk and slaughter withdrawal times are important considerations in scheduling treatment for food animals. Moreover, hospital policy must account for restricted use of certain drugs in pregnant and nursing animals because many of these animals are used for breeding.

Client education is similar to that for owners of dogs and cats; however, there should be an increased emphasis on parasite life cycles and management techniques, such as pasture rotation, to reduce parasite exposure.

Dental Care

Pets' teeth should be examined during each visit to the veterinary hospital. The veterinary technician can do the initial examination while recording the patient's history and temperature, pulse and respiration. Open the mouth or lift the animal's lips, look at the teeth and smell the breath. Depending on the veterinarian's wishes, the veterinary technician may simply make a notation regarding the condition of the teeth or may initiate a discussion with the client about regular dental care. Report to the veterinarian any dialogue that has occurred.

Ear Care

The patient's ears should be checked at each visit. The veterinary technician can perform an initial examination at the beginning of the office visit. Clients should be taught about the potential for disease and the problems that can arise from neglecting signs of ear trouble. The veterinary technician should be able to discuss the proper material to use in cleaning ears and demonstrate the proper method of ear cleaning.

Eye Care

When the chief presenting complaint is an eye problem, the veterinary technician should make ready an ophthalmoscope, eye anesthetic and fluorescein dye strips. This advanced organization is appreciated by the veterinarian and demonstrates to the client the efficiency of the staff.

Client education about the eyes can start with a puppy's or kitten's first visit to the hospital. Suggestions are given for routine eye examinations, especially when there is a breed predilection for hereditary problems. The veterinary technician should be aware of these potential hereditary eye problems.

Nutrition

The veterinary technician should weigh the patient on each visit to the hospital and compare the weight with previous ones. In mature pets, excessive variations (>10%) in weight gain or loss should be noted so that the veterinarian can explore the reasons. In immature animals, changes are expected either as the animal slims down on approaching maturity or as it gains weight with growth. Evaluate the animal's overall appearance. Does the patient appear thin, emaciated or obese? Assess the patient's overall condition in relation to its age and weight. If an adjustment in diet seems necessary, the veterinarian must be consulted.

Clients often ask the veterinary technician questions regarding diet. Information concerning nutrition is appreciated, especially on the initial visit with a puppy or a kitten. The veterinary technician should be able to discuss commercial dry, semi-moist and canned food on the basis of palatability, calories, economics, ease of feeding and balanced nutrition. Be prepared to answer questions regarding protein levels and generic versus name brands. The client may also have questions about feeding pregnant, lactating, geriatric or obese animals.

Clients often question the need for supplemental vitamins or minerals or feeding of table scraps in their pet's diet. The veterinary technician must know the veterinarian's recommendations about these additional nutritional sources.

Specialized diets for patients with diabetes mellitus or heart, liver or kidney problems must be established by the veterinarian. The technician may be asked to educate the client on dietary management of these various conditions.

Neutering Schedule for Dogs and Cats

The recommended ages for neutering surgeries vary from hospital to hospital. The guidelines given here are only suggestions. Some hospitals require a scheduled presurgical physical examination and perhaps laboratory work.

Ovariohysterectomy

Ovariohysterectomy is the proper term for the more common word, "spay." Most clients use the terms spay or neuter. You may wish to use the word ovariohysterectomy with the veterinarian and spay when talking to clients.

Dogs and cats are usually scheduled for a spay at about 6 months of age, though many veterinarians have begun doing this surgery on younger animals. This surgery is less risky when performed on a young, healthy animal.

Many doctors refuse to spay a dog if it is in estrus (heat). Blood vessels of the reproductive tract are greatly engorged and the reproductive tract is more fragile during estrus. The veterinary technician must look at the dog's vulva for signs of heat, such as swelling of the labia or a bloody vulvar discharge. If the dog appears to be in heat, speak with the veterinarian before admitting it for surgery.

Many cats presented for spay surgery are either in heat or recently pregnant. The surgery is more difficult but not to the same extent as in the dog. Most veterinarians will spay these cats, though the fee may be higher than for a standard spay.

Spaying a dog or cat in late pregnancy is more risky for the patient. Usually there is an additional fee for an ovario-hysterectomy in a pregnant animal, and the client should be advised of this fact.

Castration

Castration of dogs and cats is also known as "neutering," and the terms are frequently used interchangeably. A male cat's first hospital visit is often for neutering. Cats are often obtained when they are young kittens. A young kitten's gender is sometimes incorrectly identified. The veterinary technician should examine the genitalia of any cat admitted for neutering. Visually confirm that the cat is a male. Do not rely on the owner's belief or the cat's name.

The technician should be able to list the advantages of neutering a pet and answer clients' questions concerning weight gain and behavior changes, as well as other questions the owner may have. The fee schedule and payment policy should be memorized or readily available. Clients should be advised to make an appointment for elective surgery. Pre-surgical food and water intake, the time to arrive at the hospital, length of the usual hospital stay, suture removal (if any) and postsurgical activity recommendations should be discussed with the client.

Presurgical Considerations

When an appointment is made for surgery, the client must be informed of hospital policies regarding presurgical preparation of the patient, scheduling and payment. Typically, the surgical patient is denied access to food and water for a prescribed time before surgery. This is to minimize the possibility of vomiting and inhalation of vomitus during anesthesia. Access to water may be allowed until the time of admission.

Most hospitals require that surgical patients be current on all vaccinations. A presurgical examination is usually scheduled before admission. If the pet is receiving any medication, the veterinarian should be alerted to this fact. On admission of the animal, the client should be asked to sign a consent form for the surgery (see Chapter 5) and a written estimate of the surgical fees. Some hospitals require full payment for an elective surgery, while others may require a deposit toward the fee. Inform the owner of the anticipated length of the hospital stay.

Pet owners are usually anxious about their animal's surgery and want to know the outcome as soon as possible. Allowing time for recovery and possible delays, suggest a time for the owner to call for a progress report. Most veterinarians prefer to have the owner contact the hospital because it is less time consuming for the hospital staff. Owners will not forget to call, and they will persevere if the telephone lines are busy. Hospital staff members cannot always be that diligent.

The client's address and telephone numbers (work and home) should be checked for accuracy before admitting the pet. If a problem develops during surgery, the client should be contacted before they call for a progress report or arrive at the hospital to pick up the pet.

Most hospitals do not accept personal items, such as leads, bedding, toys or food when admitting inpatients. These items are easily misplaced, dirtied or destroyed. Finding them at the time of discharge may be time consuming. Explain that the hospital provides bedding, specialized diets and individualized care. If the owner does leave something behind, label it and place it in a prearranged place where it can be easily found.

General Postsurgical Care Instructions

When surgical patients are discharged from the hospital, the owners should be given instructions regarding surgical wound care, scheduling of followup visits, expected side effects of surgery and abnormal signs that should be reported to the hospital. Important instructions can be put in written form so that clients can refer to them over the recovery period.

The veterinary technician should discuss the effects of sedation or anesthesia, particularly if the patient is released on the same day as surgery. The pet may appear normal initially because of the excitement of departure; once home, it may act tired and unusually quiet. A prolapsed third eyelid can frighten some owners. They will be less worried if they are warned of these signs and told of the expected length of recovery.

Discharge instructions should include recommendations on feeding and providing water. Some pets are excessively thirsty following surgery. Medications are rarely necessary following elective surgery; however, if one is dispensed, the client should be taught how to administer it. Many patients do not have a bowel movement for 1-2 days after surgery because of food restrictions associated with the surgery day. Patients should be kept quiet, clean and dry during their convalescence.

Owners should be taught to perform a daily visual examination of the surgery site. Some clients wish to avoid looking at the wound, but the importance of this inspection must be emphasized. Bandages, splints or casts must be cared for, kept dry and monitored for proper fit. If absorbable sutures were used, the staff member should explain that they will gradually be absorbed by the body.

Many veterinarians prefer to reexamine their surgery patients even if absorbable sutures were used and suture removal is unnecessary. A recheck appointment can be scheduled at the time of discharge. Owners should be instructed to call the hospital before that time if any postoperative problems occur. The hospital should be notified if the patient vomits excessively, acts depressed or chews at the sutures, splint, bandage or cast. Other potential problems include bleeding from the surgery site or a foul odor from a bandage, splint or cast.

The veterinarian must establish these standard operating procedures in advance. Hospital staff members should be able to inform the client of hospital policy in clear, concise terms. When asked a similar question, the same answer should be given by each member of the staff. When you are unsure of the correct response to a client's question, consult the written hospital policy or a veterinarian before proceeding. The importance of having written SOPs cannot be overemphasized.

Recommended Reading

McCurnin D: *Clinical Textbook For Veterinary Technicians.* 2nd ed. Saunders, Philadelphia, 1990.

Pratt PW: *Medical, Surgical and Anesthetic Nursing For Veterinary Technicians.* 2nd ed. American Veterinary Publications, Goleta, CA, 1994.

Notes

2

Obtaining a History

A goal of veterinary hospitals is to provide high-quality medical care. Many things are required to meet this objective. Accurate recordkeeping is definitely one requirement. For the records to be accurate and meaningful, a complete, unbiased history must be obtained for each patient. The owner provides the past history and suggests the main problem. The veterinary technician is often primarily responsible for recording the owner's comments, asking questions to elicit more data, and observing initial actions and reactions of the patient.

Basic Information

Basic information about the client and the patient is always included in a medical record. Basic data may be recorded by a receptionist before the veterinary technician sees the patient for the first time. This information is necessary to establish identity and some baseline data for future reference.

Client Information

The basic data include the owner's name, address and telephone number. Accuracy is important. Review these data for clients who have not been seen recently. Names, addresses and telephone numbers are often changed. Obtain business as well as home telephone numbers. In cases of emergency while the animal is hospitalized, access to a business phone number could be extremely important.

Patient Information

Other basic information includes the patient's name, species, breed and sex. The call name of purebred animals is preferred to the registered name. For example, a dog may respond to Joe, but not to Abercrombies Jocoby's Prize. Make note of any degree or title (example: show champion) earned by the animal. This is valuable information for the veterinarian and the veterinary technician about the patient's past activities, its value and possibly the owner's feelings for it.

If the animal has been neutered, the appropriate abbreviation or symbol should be affixed to the statement of gender. The symbol Mc or X denotes a castrated male, while Fs or the symbol X+ denotes a spayed female.

The patient's age at the time of the initial visit is recorded. This is not changed with each trip to the hospital. Instead, the veterinarian adds the elapsed months or years to the first recorded age. Recording the date of birth also may be helpful.

Finally, the animal's weight is recorded as part of the basic information. The weight should be determined at each visit to document any drastic changes. If the weight change is alarming, body weight can be monitored more closely. The weight is also used to calculate drug doses, so accuracy is important.

Communication Skills

General Principles

To get an accurate and unbiased history from the owner, the veterinary technician must be skillful in the use of words as well as in observing the client's body language. To establish the required confidence level, be sincere. Sincerity can be projected in a variety of ways, including body language, voice and mannerisms. Eye contact with owners is important to encourage their confidence in you. People put a great deal of trust in someone who will "look them in the eye." Concentrate on this skill until it becomes easy. At the same time, note how many other people cannot or will not maintain eye contact with you. What are your reactions to these people?

Use the patient's name in conversation, and touch the patient in light, easy movements. These actions do not go unnoticed by the owner. Clients think positively of a staff member who cares enough to learn the patient's name and who demonstrates a friendly rapport with the animal. The result may be a more revealing history. Also, the personal touch and pleasant voice may help to quiet a fractious patient.

Asking Questions

When obtaining a history and speaking to clients, remember that each client is an individual. Try to assess the client's general intelligence, education and social background, and then adjust your language accordingly.

Adjust your discussion to suit the client. For example, you might use more scientific terms and a generally higher level of discussion with a highly educated person, such as a physician or an engineer, than with a person of limited education. Do not, however, "talk down" to or patronize a person of lesser intelligence or education. Regardless of a client's apparent educational level and background, always be professional, polite and pleasant. Do not use profanity and "street talk."

Use neutral statements when asking questions. The questions should be broad and open ended so that the owner has a chance to give unbiased answers. Don't ask leading questions. Here's an example of a leading question and a more appropriately phrased question:

Leading Question: "Is your pet drinking a great deal of water?" In this case, the question could make the owner feel that his or her pet should be drinking a great deal of water. Also, the answer could easily be a very short yes or no. These types of answers do not add much to the data base.

Better Question: "Can you tell me about your pet's water consumption?" With this question you have not prejudiced the owner's thoughts. There is no suggestion that water consumption should be great or small. Also, the answer to this kind of question will be more descriptive than a cursory yes or no.

Be alert to an owner's answers that require more elaboration. Further questioning may be necessary to generate greater detail. For example:

Owner: "My dog drinks at least 2 bowls of water each day."

Technician: "How many cups of water does the bowl hold?"

In obtaining a history, establish a routine and try not to deviate from it. If you develop a standard routine in obtaining a history, the history-taking procedure will require less time and important questions will not be omitted. The established routine can vary slightly, but try to develop a sequence that is comfortable and practical.

The Owner's Responses

It requires some skill to obtain an accurate, unbiased history from most owners. A few clients are excellent observers; they may even have had training in observation. Others have not paid attention to their animal's activities, so an accurate history is impossible. Still others may purposely withhold information because they are ashamed of their pet's condition, lack of confidence in you or they have personality quirks.

Information from very young owners or very old owners may be unreliable. Clients in these age groups may not comprehend the significance of each question. Your evaluation must be especially astute with these groups. You must realize when facts have been omitted and then attempt to extract more information.

Remember that the owner has an opinion concerning his or her pet's health. Respect that opinion and resist the temptation to belittle the owner. For example:

Owner: "I think my dog has distemper."

Technician: "I doubt it. Please let the veterinarian make the diagnosis!"

Such responses alienate the client and make an accurate history more difficult to obtain. Any rapport that you may have developed with the owner can be destroyed with such a careless remark.

Recording the History

Main Complaint

After you obtain or verify the basic information on the chart, establish the main reason for the office visit. Start your questioning this way. Record the main complaint as clinical signs, not as a diagnosis. For example, the major complaint is "vomiting and diarrhea." These are clinical signs. Recording "bacterial gastroenteritis" would signify a diagnosis that could be incorrect.

The next step is to ascertain and record the duration of signs. In our example, quizzing the owner elicits the fact that vomiting and diarrhea have been occurring for 12 hours. Thus, the duration of signs is noted as 12 hours.

Present Complaint

The most logical sequence of questioning is to begin with the present complaint. Because there are many possible complaints, you could have a variety of outlines to follow in gathering information, depending upon the signs. Record all information sequentially and start with the most recent date. This may be difficult with certain owners, but try to elicit information from the onset of the current complaint to as far back as they can remember.

During this discussion, you may need to ask additional questions, especially when certain key points need elaboration. Establish the exact onset of signs and any preceding exposure to sick animals. Determine if other animals or people in contact with the patient developed a similar illness, especially if you suspect an infectious or zoonotic disease.

Ascertain if the current illness is unique to this animal or if it is merely one in a series of similar episodes. If the condition is a recurrent one, obtain information about previous dates and duration of illness and treatments.

Past History

Make a point of requesting the information on the past history of the patient. For patients with established medical records, questions about the past history often elicit new information about previous major illnesses, accidents, allergies and surgeries. Review and update the data if necessary in these categories.

A complete history of immunizations, with dates, is valuable to the veterinarian. This information may already be in the medical record from previous visits. However, if major time blocks are unaccounted for, this suggests involvement of other veterinarians, and questions on immunizations are necessary.

For new patients, information about previous illnesses is very important, especially the dates, diagnoses, treatments and any resulting complications. If the animal has not had previous problems, note this so that the veterinarian will realize that the question was raised.

A history of allergies may influence the veterinarian's selection of treatment and medication. Previous accidents and surgeries could be important in choice of laboratory tests and interpretation of laboratory data or radiographs. Radiography may be important if there is a history of road trauma or orthopedic surgery.

Record any information on the parents of the patient and the health of the parents, siblings or offspring. This type of information, if available, is sometimes helpful in diagnosis. Hereditary conditions, in particular, can be diagnosed based on a history of near relatives. For example:

Owner: "The parents of this dog had hip dysplasia. Could my dog's lameness be caused by hip dysplasia?"

Finally, remember to record information on diet, shelter, grooming and medication. Each of these items could be helpful to the veterinarian evaluating the case.

Temperature, Pulse and Respiration

In some hospitals, veterinary technicians must record the temperature and pulse and respiration rates (TPR) for each patient. This routine examination can be done easily in less than 5 minutes. Concentrate during the pulse and respiration phases to get accurate readings.

System Review

A veterinary technician is not a veterinarian and is neither expected, required nor licensed to render a diagnosis. This does not mean that the technician should not observe and record normal and abnormal patient data. Notes and questions for the attending veterinarian are appreciated and may help the veterinarian to concentrate on abnormal findings.

Body openings include the eyes, nose, mouth, ears, vulva, prepuce and anus. Look for discharges, odors and growths from body openings as you record the TPR. Record any head tilt, loss of hair, irritated skin, edema, effusions, limb or joint swelling and lameness.

A cough, pain when touched, and even soft feces observed on the thermometer should elicit questions for the owner. Small signs can lead to more information and possibly aid the veterinarian in establishing a diagnosis. Be inquisitive;

record signs, but allow the veterinarian to pursue important findings.

The recorded history, observations made by both the veterinarian and the technician, and the veterinarian's physical examination of the patient contribute to the diagnosis. When the diagnosis is unclear or needs confirmation, the veterinarian may order clinical laboratory tests. The veterinary technician is often responsible for specimen collection, and performing and recording these tests. Try to anticipate the veterinarian's needs by preparing the necessary equipment for specimen collection.

The composite picture of patient history, physical observations and laboratory test results usually leads to a diagnosis. The ability of the veterinary technician to obtain a complete and accurate history is important.

For Review and Discussion

1. What data are considered to be the basic information in a patient's history?

2. Practice using neutral questions.

3. In obtaining histories, establishing a routine is important. What routine would you follow?

4. Why is the main complaint listed as a sign?

Recommended Reading

Freeland F: The problem-oriented medical record. *Vet Technician* 9:132-137, 1988.

Langham M: Medical records for hospital patients. *Vet Technician* 5:297-303, 1984.

Stegdale L: The problem-oriented medical record for veterinary practice. *Compan Anim Pract* 1: 901-913, 1984.

Notes

3

Management of Emergencies

Some telephone calls to a veterinary practice are made in the event of true emergencies. This is evident by the seriousness of the injury or illness described or by the demeanor of the caller. With other calls, it may be difficult to determine whether this is truly an emergency situation. A combination of common sense and experience dictates what cases are emergencies or potential emergencies. Because you may have had little clinical experience in deciding which cases constitute true emergencies, the choice can be a difficult one.

General Principles

An emergency is a sudden occurrence that demands immediate action. Many conditions are serious and require immediate attention. You should be aware of these and, using common sense and experience, recognize and react to them.

Certainly, when a critical choice must be made, consultation with the veterinarian is necessary. Conversely, many emergencies are so obvious that continual dialogue with the doctor can shake the confidence the veterinarian has in your decision-making abilities.

Some suspected emergencies turn out not to be emergencies. The animal's condition is stable and immediate care is not crucial. Veterinarians will not question your abilities if you err in favor of early intervention. If, on the other hand, you do not recognize an emergency, thereby allowing the problem to worsen, the client will question the reputation and ability of the veterinarian because you represent the hospital and the professional staff.

Clients may have their own definition of an emergency. To some owners, diarrhea in their dog is an emergency, while to other clients it is only an inconvenience and a minor problem. If you cannot persuade the client that the situation is not serious, treat the call as an emergency. When this scenario develops, express your true thoughts and feelings to the veterinarian before the animal's arrival. In this way, colleagues will not criticize you for "crying wolf."

There will be times when the veterinary technician is alone at the clinic and a client calls in with a true emergency. If the veterinarian is unavailable, refer the client to an emergency care facility (if one exists) or to a nearby veterinarian. Knowledge of area veterinarians and their addresses and telephone numbers is essential. You may need to call another hospital for the client. Giving first aid instructions to the owner may be life saving.

Be as much help as you can. At all times remain calm, though the caller may not be. Positive, definitive, confident instructions from you may alleviate the client's distress.

Sometimes a critically ill patient is presented to the hospital without advance notice, when the veterinarian is unavailable. In this case, the veterinary technician should assess the problem. Another hospital staff member should call the veterinarian to notify him or her of the situation and obtain further instructions. Ideally, the hospital has written protocols for treatment of certain emergency conditions. An example might be heatstroke, occurring when a dog has been closed in a car during the summer. The protocol could list some typical clinical signs, such as body temperature exceeding 105 F, convulsions or possible coma, and dyspnea.

The written standard operating procedure (SOP) would list sequentially the steps for treatment of hyperthermia. With such a protocol, the veterinary technician can give emergency care and is considered to be under the supervision of a veterinarian. The veterinarian can then advise further treatment via telephone, based on the technician's observations.

If the veterinarian cannot be reached, the technician should attempt to stabilize the animal's condition while someone else calls a neighboring veterinarian to refer the patient. In the absence of a written protocol, the technician should administer only life-saving first aid, such as direct pressure on a bleeding wound. Refer the animal to another veterinarian. Help the client by calling the referral veterinarian and explaining the situation. Give written travel directions to the owner or take the patient to the other hospital yourself. The positive public relations realized can be immeasurable. You have demonstrated your care and concern.

Common Emergency Conditions

Common emergencies include massive hemorrhage, penetrating wounds to the abdomen or thorax, coma or loss of consciousness, ingestion of a known or suspected poison, massive musculoskeletal injuries, respiratory embarrassment and shock.

Emergencies can also occur within the hospital. The wards are filled with sick animals and surgical patients who can develop cardiac arrest, suffer an anaphylactic reaction or develop acute bacteremia or toxemia. Technicians working in a hospital are required to administer basic first aid and must be able to give cardiopulmonary resuscitation (CPR) or describe the techniques to clients calling by telephone.

Contacting the Veterinarian

In equine or food animal practices, the veterinarian is often on farm visits when a client calls. You must then contact the veterinarian at the farm site or on the practice vehicle's mobile telephone. Make sure you have the first and last name of the caller, a telephone number and the address. If you are unfamiliar with the name, get directions to their farm. The caller may be a new client or the veterinarian may be new to the practice and may not know the farm's location.

Some large animal veterinarians have a 2-way radio system in their vehicle. You may need to learn how to operate the home base system. Many now have cellular telephones. If there is no answer, the veterinarian may be out of the vehicle and in the barn. In this case, or if the veterinarian does not have a 2-way radio or vehicle telephone, you must telephone the farms the veterinarian is visiting so as to relay the emergency message.

The hospital staff must keep a list of farm visits for each day, the order of those visits and the estimated time for each. Telephone numbers can be looked up if necessary, but if the basic scheduling information is not available, trying to contact the veterinarian will be both frustrating and unproductive.

If you leave a message for the veterinarian, make sure that all the information is correct and complete. An animal's life may be at stake, as well as a farmer's income. If you are concerned that the message may not be delivered properly, ask that the veterinarian call you back immediately upon arriving at the farm. In this way you can deliver the message yourself.

Remember that you are not rendering a diagnosis when you must decide if a situation represents a true emergency. Rather, you are evaluating the history and the signs described by the owner. The situation may or may not turn out to be as serious as suspected. However, if the caller is describing a true emergency, you should err in favor of caution. A diagnosis is a decision based on examination, observation and facts. Your belief that a situation represents an emergency is an opinion and an estimation of what seems probable.

For Review and Discussion

1. What key items must you obtain from the caller in establishing that a problem is a true emergency?

2. Discuss probable emergencies in dogs and cats.

3. Discuss probable emergencies in horses and cattle.

Recommended Reading

McCurnin D: *Clinical Textbook For Veterinary Technicians.* 2nd ed. Saunders, Philadelphia, 1990.

28   *Chapter 3*

Pratt PW: *Medical, Surgical and Anesthetic Nursing For Veterinary Technicians.* 2nd ed. American Veterinary Publications, Goleta, CA, 1994.

Notes

4

Scheduling

Operating an efficient veterinary hospital requires successful management of many facets of the business, including smooth, workable office hours and surgical procedures. Scheduling daily office hours and surgery would seem at first glance to be easy. Indeed, it would be easy if clients arrived on time, if every client had an appointment and if there were no emergencies. This rarely happens.

Whether or not scheduling office hours and surgical procedures is in your job description, you should understand the basics of scheduling and be able to perform it should the need arise.

Scheduling Client Visits

Some hospitals see patients only by appointment, while others use a first-come, first-served walk-in arrangement. An appointment-only policy is impractical in practices with a small caseload or in mixed practices with a limited number of days or hours for small animal clients. The appointment-only plan maintains structured office hours with predetermined staff, rooms and appointment time limits. This type of arrangement works best for the predominantly small animal hospital with a clientele accustomed to services by appointment. Generally, "by appointment only" requires more planning but results in less waiting for the client.

Staffing for appointments depends on the size of the practice and the time of day. A rule of thumb is that one veterinary technician is assigned to each veterinarian. Usually there is one receptionist for every 2-3 veterinarians on duty. With an increasing number of veterinarians handling office hours, there must be an increasing number of receptionists to handle admissions, payments and the ever-present telephone.

It is most efficient to assign 2 examination rooms to each veterinarian handling office hours. In 1 room, a veterinary technician can take a history from the client, record the pet's temperature, pulse and respiration (TPR), and collect laboratory samples from the patient. At the same time, in a second examination room, the veterinarian can review data or decide on treatment for another patient.

The time allotted to an office call is commonly 15 minutes, but policies vary. Most patient needs can be met in 15 minutes. A few patients may require less time, while some need more than the allotted time. These patients should not be slighted because a predetermined, arbitrary time has elapsed. When scheduling office hours, attempt to balance the time slots so that the veterinarian remains busy and the appointments are as punctual as possible, thereby giving the appearance of an efficient, professional health team.

Appointments that usually take less than 15 minutes include nail clips, suture removals, cast or splint rechecks, blood or other sample collection, and rechecks of previously diagnosed conditions. Some appointments require 2 or more time slots, for 30 or more minutes, such as complex cases referred to the hospital by another veterinarian and multi-pet appointments. Any patient that requires sedation will need additional office time. Finally, it makes good business sense to spend additional time with first-time patients. This is because of the many basic questions that are commonly discussed and the need to establish a veterinarian-client bond.

Some cases can disrupt a perfectly constructed schedule. Examples include an undiagnosed sick animal showing central nervous system signs, a lame patient, and a patient with dietary or behavior problems. These patients take longer to see, they infringe on the next appointment and they disrupt the routine, but they are an important part of veterinary practice.

The appointment schedule may be preserved when the veterinarian recognizes that a patient requires further laboratory testing or radiographs for a proper diagnosis. Early recognition that hospitalization, testing and medical treatment are necessary may get the schedule back to normal. Then, just as the professional staff begins to breathe easy again, the office is besieged by a series of emergencies. Scheduling is not always easy!

Traditional appointment books indicate the time slots with a space for the client's last name, the patient's species and name, and the principal complaint (Fig 1). Each veterinarian in a multi-doctor practice may have an appointment book.

The client's telephone numbers can also be included. If the appointment must be changed or postponed because of an unforeseen problem, it saves time to have the telephone number in the appointment book. Telephone numbers are also available from the records if patient records are pulled before their arrival, except for first-time patients.

When setting up the schedule, get enough information from the client to retrieve records or initiate a new record. However, space in the appointment book is generally limited, so a complete description of the problem is not possible. The principal complaint (eg, lameness) should be listed; this aids the scheduling process and alerts the medical team to possible problems and tests the patient may require.

As an example, Dr. Adams is using 2 rooms and 2 veterinary technicians to their full capabilities. The veterinary technicians obtain a TPR and a history before the doctor enters the room. Dr. Adams devotes full attention to the client and leaves restraint of the patient to the veterinary technician. The veterinarian is involved in diagnosis, treat-

Figure 1. Example of a companion animal appointment book. The 10:15, 10:45 and 11:15 appointments were not filled because Jones, Corpora and Loring will require longer than 15 minutes.

	Dr. Adams	
	Room 1	Room 2
10:00	Jones A – cat, Paul, first visit	Smith B – cat, Lefty, cast
10:15	" "	VanZandt V – dog, Spot, lame
10:30	Harding C – dog, Gomer, diarrhea	Corpora P – dog, Browney, behavior problem
10:45	Samuels J – dog, Sam, coughing	" "
11:00	Loring L – dog, Suzie, referred by Mrs. Callahan	Anderson T – dog, Jesse, suture removal
11:15	" "	Adams E – dog, Pete, nail clip

ment decisions and prognosis. Prescription filling, many of the instructions and client education are delegated to the veterinary technician. The receptionist collects the fee while the veterinary technician prepares the room for the next patient.

By organizing the staff as a health team with well-defined responsibilities, Dr. Adams can see more than the minimum of 4 clients per hour. Proper staff use increases the case volume of the hospital without extending office hours. As time demands on the veterinarian increase, full use of staff is important for efficient veterinary hospital management.

Guidelines for Scheduling Client Visits

When scheduling outpatient appointments, decide how much time the patient will need and attempt to schedule accordingly. If you believe the problem is complicated, block out 2 time slots. Try to combine a short visit with another short appointment. On a busy day, schedule 2 short appointments, such as suture removals, for the same time.

In our example the veterinarian is using 2 rooms for office visits. A third room could be available for emergencies or, if appointments are backing up, to alleviate a congested reception area.

If possible, group appointments early in the day. This is the time when staff members are rested and ready to go. Scheduling appointments intermittently throughout office hours is not an efficient use of time.

There are slow periods in all veterinary hospitals. Though they may be pleasant respites for you, they are not welcomed by your employer. On slow days, consolidate appointments by grouping them together as much as possible. This gives the clients the favorable impression that the practice is busy and thriving. Consolidating appointments makes the entire hospital staff more efficient as well.

When scheduling appointments, leave a few slots open later in the day. If office hours are from 1 pm to 6 pm, leave some openings between 5 pm and 6 pm. Clients who observe their animals' illnesses in the afternoon will want the animal examined that evening. If all the late appointments are already taken, there will be no open times for these emergencies, and the staff will have to stay at the hospital past closing time to take care of these cases.

There are other elements to take into account. In multi-veterinarian practices, some clients prefer to see a particular veterinarian. They may be personal friends or social acquaintances, or the client may have more confidence in a particular veterinarian. Whenever possible, these clients' wishes should be recognized and accommodated.

Other clients may request a particular appointment time because of a transportation problem or a busy schedule. Sometimes their request cannot be easily met. Give these clients the benefit of the doubt and make an effort, within reason, to accommodate them.

Occasionally, while you are talking to a client to set up an appointment, you will suspect an emergency situation that the client does not recognize. For example, the client may wish to bring in a tom cat tomorrow because of suspected constipation. The history and description suggest a possible urinary obstruction, an emergency situation requiring immediate treatment. Without rendering a diagnosis, try to convince the client that an earlier veterinary examination is prudent. Any suspected serious condition should be investigated as soon as possible.

Doctors also have preferences that must be considered when scheduling office hours. In a multi-veterinarian hospital, one veterinarian may be more expert with cage birds, another with horses, and another with orthopedic cases. Also, most veterinarians prefer to see and evaluate their previous surgical or medical patients.

When you are on the telephone scheduling an office visit, remember not to tie up the telephone for an unnecessarily long time. Obtain the basic information, such as owner's name, address and telephone numbers, the patient species and name or identification number, last visit to the hospital (if any), and a brief description of the problem. Details of the situation can be gathered when the client arrives.

Scheduling appointments for farm visits is on a looser structure. Instead of a specific appointment time, set up the farm visit for a general time during a specific day. If possible, group visits to farms in one area in the same day. During spring and fall herd work, a veterinarian may go to only 1 or 2 farms a day, especially if the herds are large.

Scheduling Surgical Procedures

Elective surgeries are often scheduled for the morning hours, when the surgical team is fresh. This timing allows patients to recover completely from anesthesia while the hospital is fully staffed. Clients can call or be called about their animal's condition as early in the day as possible. Some veterinarians choose to do elective surgeries, such as ovariohysterectomies and castrations, only on certain days of the week.

Busy practices, with limited surgical room space, may schedule surgery throughout the day. Some surgeons prefer a morning schedule, while others prefer an afternoon schedule. It is also possible that the team will need to work all day to complete all surgeries.

An important factor in scheduling surgery is the type of procedure to be done. While most veterinarians do all types of surgery, some veterinarians specialize in eye surgery, orthopedics or soft tissue surgery. You must know the type of surgery to be done, the client's preference of surgeon, the surgeon's specialty, if any, and the time the surgeon is available.

Some surgery is classified as "dirty" surgery. Examples include a horse with a 4-day-old laceration, a dog hit by a car, and a cat with contaminated fight wounds. Also, a dog with porcupine quills in its muzzle requires sedation, a treatment room, equipment and a portion of the surgical team. Dirty surgery can be performed in a room other than the surgical suite. Perhaps only the cold sterilization tray is needed, rather than an autoclaved surgical pack. The staff member doing the surgical scheduling must keep these variables in mind while juggling rooms, equipment and professional staff.

Competent and sufficient help must be available for surgery. A veterinary technician can administer premedications, and induce and monitor anesthesia. A circulating veterinary technician to prep and position the patient, and to open drapes and surgical packs is helpful. The veterinarian may also need someone to assist in the surgery.

Someone is needed to clean and autoclave the instruments for the next surgery. The surgical suite and operating table must be cleaned and sanitized; drapes and gowns must be soaked and washed. These jobs can be done by a single full-time veterinary technician or several part-time technicians. Surgery should be scheduled so that the veterinarian is kept busy, assistance is always available, surgery is not delayed waiting for sterilized instruments, and the patient is given the best care possible.

How many surgical packs are available? Are the general instrument packs suitable for any type of surgery? Does the hospital have an orthopedic or an ophthalmic surgical pack? How long will it take to clean, repack and autoclave instruments? These are all considerations when scheduling surgery.

Successful scheduling also requires knowledge of the time needed to complete the more common surgeries, such as canine and feline ovariohysterectomy and castration, cesarean section and bone pinning. Develop a list of common surgical procedures and the time required for each. When creating this list, consider the experience and speed of each veterinarian in the practice. New graduate veterinarians take much more time in surgery than experienced surgeons.

With knowledge of available help, the surgeon and the type of surgery, you can become adept at creating a surgery schedule. This is without factoring in the emergencies that always seem to appear just when you think it is safe to order your pizza for lunch. Your reputation for arranging smooth office hours and surgery is earned by giving attention to detail and allowing for flexibility with regard to unexpected interruptions.

For Review and Discussion

1. What is the "rule of thumb" for the number of veterinary technicians and receptionists needed when 3 veterinarians are conducting office hours concurrently?

2. List as many examples as possible of office hour appointments that would take less than 15 minutes of the doctor's time.

3. One veterinarian is doing surgery with 2 sterile surgical packs. It takes 30 minutes to clean, repack and autoclave each set of instruments. The veterinarian can routinely do

a dog spay in 30 minutes, a bone pinning in 45 minutes, a cat spay in 20 minutes and a dog castration in 20 minutes. The veterinarian wants to start surgery at 9 am and go to a luncheon meeting at noon. There will be a 10-minute break between surgeries to position animals and rescrub. The veterinarian has 1 dog castration, 1 dog spay, 1 cat spay and 1 bone pinning. Schedule the surgeries so they are completed before noon and there is a fresh, sterile pack for each procedure.

Recommended Reading

Colville T, in Pratt PW: *Medical, Surgical and Anesthetic Nursing For Veterinary Technicians.* 2nd ed. American Veterinary Publications, Goleta, CA, 1994.

McCurnin D: *Veterinary Hospital Management.* Lippincott, Philadelphia, 1988.

Notes

5

Records and Recordkeeping

Accurate recordkeeping is essential to the operation of a veterinary hospital. Hospital staff members must have a thorough understanding of the records required in a clinic, the importance of accuracy and completeness, and the reasons for keeping records. Every facet of the hospital's day-to-day operation involves record keeping. No one on the hospital staff is excluded from maintaining records of their activity.

Legal Issues

All veterinary hospitals and research facilities maintain records, though not every facility has the same type of records. Each hospital determines the records it requires and the manner in which to maintain them. All research institutions and an increasing number of veterinary hospitals are using computers for record keeping.

There are many types of records and formats. The medicolegal requirements vary in each state, but records are legal documents and therefore are subject to subpoena and are admissible as evidence in a court of law. Examples of when records might be used in court include insurance claims, animal injury claims and malpractice claims.

Handwritten records must be legible and accurate. They must be done in permanent ink. If errors occur when establishing a record, they should be crossed out and the corrections made, dated and initialed by the person making the entry.

Complete obliteration or erasure of the original record would suggest to a court that tampering was attempted by the hospital staff. To prevent this interpretation, a single line through the error is recommended.

Certain records and consent forms may require the client's signature. Do not allow a minor to sign, as a minor cannot legally enter into a contract.

Record Ownership

The owner of the records is the veterinary practice, not the client. The client has purchased the service and information contained in a record; however, the client does not own the original records. Medical records include, but are not limited to, laboratory results, electrocardiogram (ECG) tracings, radiographs and medical treatment reports.

This means that hospital staff members must not release records, photocopies of records or even pertinent information to the client or agent of the client unless specifically permitted to do so by the attending veterinarian or the practice owner. The original records are a legal document and must be retained by the practice. Release of this information is at the discretion of the veterinarian or practice owner.

A client may move and change veterinarians or consult with or be referred to another veterinarian. Any request for transfer of records should be in writing so that the veterinarian can authorize the release. Usually, an abstract is prepared of the medical information. The client is rarely giving a photocopy of the original record. They should not be allowed to review the original record without the veterinarian's permission because they may not be able to interpret all the entries, and a misunderstanding could result. By reviewing the records and recording the important and necessary information, the veterinarian provides the necessary data for the next veterinarian and retains the original legal document. The best procedure is to mail the prepared records to the new veterinarian, rather than to give them to the client.

Certain medical records, such as radiographs, are also helpful to a referral veterinarian. These items are often loaned to the referral veterinarian. Hospital staff members who receive borrowed records may be required to maintain and eventually return them.

Confidentiality

The professional staff must understand that the information contained in all medical records is confidential. The client's privacy must be protected. There should be no discussion of the records with outside parties without the client's written permission. An exception is in court, where the hospital staff cannot refuse to give testimony regarding privileged communication with a client.

Another exception to the general confidentiality statement is the requirement of local, state and federal agencies to report certain contagious and zoonotic diseases. This reporting is done by the veterinarian. Information about the client or their animal(s) may be requested by the agency. In this circumstance, hospital staff may have to supply otherwise confidential information. An example would be revealing a dog's rabies vaccination status to the County Health Officer following that animal's exposure to rabies.

Statute of Limitations

Records must be legally retained for a certain time. This period varies from state to state but usually is 7 years from the date of the last visit or discharge. Most hospital records are maintained at least that long. Often, hospital policy dictates that inactive cases (over 3 years since the last visit) are purged from the current files and placed in an inactive file. If a patient does eventually return to the practice, it is possible to find their records. Filing space can be a problem in any practice and inactive records can be removed yearly. Store active files in one area that is easily accessible to both the veterinarian and the staff. Inactive files should also be accessible to all; however, they are typically kept in less central areas of the hospital.

After the statute of limitations has expired (7 years), the records can be destroyed. To maintain confidentiality, the best policy is to burn or shred them. They should not be discarded without proper defacing.

The introduction of computerized records has increased storage capabilities. Staff members must know how to access computerized records quickly. Current computer programs for medical records are designed mostly for basic data on the owner, the patient's vaccination records and client billing. Some hospitals also may require the daily addition (input) of case histories, laboratory results or other data on treatment and diagnosis.

Storing and Filing Medical Records

There are many medical record filing systems. Most medical records are arranged alphabetically by the owner's last name (Fig 1). Each patient is given an individual record and, in the case of multiple pets, the animals' records are arranged alphabetically.

Some systems are arranged numerically, with a case number for either the client or the patient.

Color coding is another increasingly common filing system. In this system, each letter of the alphabet is given a colored tab. Misfiling is easier to prevent and identify because the record can be visually appraised. Finding files should be a quick and easy job.

Despite everyone's best efforts, records can be lost. Incorrect filing, misspelled names and misplaced records do occasionally occur. Not only is this embarrassing to the hospital staff, it is also stressful for the veterinarian and inconve-

Figure 1. Alphabetic ordering of client and patient names.

Owner's Name	Patient's Name
Butler, William	Mickey
Buttignol, Stan	Joe
Callihan, Lorin	Dean
Callihan, Lorin	Sammy

nient to the owner. If a record is lost, explain the situation to the client and continue to search for it. Begin a new record immediately. In addition to input from the client and veterinarian, you may be able to add data from radiography, laboratory and vaccination log books.

Medical Records

Log Books

Log books can be used in any part of a hospital. These books contain entries of services provided. Log books are usually bound separately and kept in the appropriate area of the hospital. Examples of possible log books include radiography, surgery, euthanasia, laboratory, use of controlled drugs and necropsy logs.

Log books contain a potentially valuable data collection. Some figures obtainable from a laboratory log might be the number of heartworm examinations done in a particular year or the volume of heartworm blood checks in the month of May, as compared with other months. This information can be used to determine when to send out reminder cards or whether or not to order additional heartworm supplies for May. Log book data can also help to determine the production and profitability of a certain department. For example, how many radiographs were made in the past year? Would the addition of an automatic processor be practical, based on this volume?

Finally, log books are required by law when dispensing controlled drugs, such as barbiturates and narcotics. A record must be kept of the use of these drugs, the owner and patient, the amount used and a current inventory (Fig 2).

Special forms are required for ordering controlled drugs (Fig 3). Purchase of controlled drugs, such as barbiturates and narcotics, requires a special license from the Drug Enforcement Administration. When the drugs arrive, the

Figure 2. Sample log sheet for thiamylal.

	Drug: Thiamylal sodium		
Total	**Description**	**ml used**	**ml remaining**
3/1/94	Mixed 5g thiamylal, 4% solution	—	125
3/1/94	Gaynor K, dog Bitsy	5	120
3/2/94	Lossing W, dog Petey	7	113
3/2/94	Debray M, dog Honey	10	103
3/2/94	Cummings T, dog Ajax	12	91

Figure 3. Official form for ordering controlled substances.

invoice and the actual drug must match. The drugs are kept under lock and key. Double-locked areas (a safe within a safe) are necessary for storage of narcotics. The special order forms are also secured in the safe.

Medical Records of Animals

The most common records kept in a hospital are the medical records of animals. These records must be individualized with a separate record for each animal. They must be complete and accurate. In all cases, they contain certain basic information: the owner's name, address and telephone numbers; and the patient's name, species, age, sex, breed, and color. In addition, the information includes the date the patient is seen, the chief complaint, history, clinical signs, diagnosis, prognosis, authorization records, radiographic data, laboratory reports, and vaccination and surgical records.

Financial information is often included in veterinary medical records. The fee charged, the amount paid and the balance are examples of financial information. However, separate billing is preferable and is becoming a more common practice. This separates the business and medical aspects of a practice. Separating out the financial information generates more paperwork and initial input, but it eliminates the clutter in a medical record and is less time consuming in the long term.

Two basic formats are used in animal medical records. The most popular is the *chronologic method,* in which the events are entered as they occur (Fig 4).

The second method is *problem oriented.* This method is used mostly in teaching institutions but is being adapted by private practitioners. It is more involved than the conventional method because each medical problem is identified, along with a specific treatment plan and treatment results (Fig 5).

Vaccination Records

Vaccination records list the type of vaccine used, such as canine or feline distemper, rabies, hepatitis, leptospirosis, parvovirus, feline respiratory diseases and feline leukemia virus. The patient's basic data are recorded on the vaccination record. The forms are usually provided by the vaccine's manufacturer. They must be completed correctly and promptly. The forms are made out in triplicate. The original is given to the client at the time of vaccination and 1 copy

Figure 4. Example of a chronologic medical record.

3/20/94 am	Diarrhea, Temp. 101.5, Pulse 75, Resp. – Panting. Fecal sample taken. Diathal 0.2 ml. Hospitalized.
3/20/94 pm	One loose stool – no blood. Fecal negative for parasites. Eating, drinking, temp. 101.5.

Figure 5. Example of a problem-oriented medical record.

Problems	Treatment, Tests
Dermatitis	Rule out possibility of mange, check for hypothyroidism. Skin scraping, T3-4, cholesterol level.
Impacted anal sacs	Relieve impaction, manual expression, flush anal sacs with saline.
Long nails	Clip nails.

becomes part of the medical record. The third copy often becomes the vaccination reminder, which is sent to the client when the next vaccination is due.

Vaccination Reminders

Vaccination reminders are sent out as necessary, usually yearly. Keeping patients current on their vaccinations is important for disease prevention. Sending notices to clients is ethical and beneficial for the client, animal and practitioner. Clients learn to expect and depend on timely vaccination reminders. The response to vaccination reminders produces a large portion of a practice's income. Most important, preventing disease is preferable to treating disease. Large animal practitioners can also use vaccination reminders for their clients' herds or flocks.

The reminder system is often set up on a computer program, making the third vaccination record copy unnecessary except as a tool for computer entry. Whether or not the hospital is computerized, it is important to keep the medical records current. It is very poor public relations when a client whose pet died of kidney failure in January receives a vaccination reminder for a distemper booster in April.

Neutering Certificates

Proof of spaying or castration may be necessary to obtain reduced licensing fees for dogs. The canine licensing fee may be much reduced for an altered patient. Currently, in most states, cat owners are not subject to a licensing fee. The blank certificate forms are often obtained from a drug distributor or a commercial printer (Fig 6). They usually consist of an original, which goes to the client, and a tab, which is retained by the hospital.

These certificates often need replacement, as clients commonly lose them before licensing their pet. Replacing certificates can be a time-consuming part of your daily tasks. Here are some tips to prevent this:

- Make sure the owner receives a neutering certificate when the patient goes home.
- Make sure the owner knows the significance and importance of the certificate, *ie,* a reduced license fee.
- Number the certificates and keep a list of the numbers and the owner's name. Cross filing makes it much easier to find the name, date and surgeon when certificate replacement is necessary.

Euthanasia Consent Forms

Forms authorizing euthanasia of an animal can be purchased, or they may be provided by some drug distributors

Figure 6. Sample neutering certificate.

RETAIN THIS CERTIFICATE

Certificate of Spaying

THIS IS TO CERTIFY, that I have performed an ovario-hysterectomy this ....

day of ....on a female dog of the following description:

Name.................................Breed.................Age...............Color...................

Belonging to...

Whose address is...

No...................................   --
                                        VETERINARIAN

(Fig 7). A consent form should be filled out before any euthanasia. The form gives the veterinarian permission to euthanize the animal. In this way, the client cannot claim later that permission was not given.

The euthanasia form states that the animal has not bitten anyone in the previous 10 days. This is because, if the animal were a rabies suspect and had bitten someone in the previous 10 days, examination of its brain, after euthanasia, would be required to determine if the person bitten had to undergo rabies treatment.

The owner or their designated representative must sign the form. The staff member who helps prepare the form should initial it in case the veterinarian has any questions.

There are times when the owner or the owner's agent is not present but euthanasia is requested, such as for a hospitalized, terminally ill patient. If the veterinarian permits the client's verbal authorization for euthanasia, a hospital staff member *should* make sure the owner understands what euthanasia is and what is going to happen. There can be no mistakes here. Attempt to get the owner to come to the

Figure 7. Sample euthanasia consent form.

Date:_____

I give the Delaware Animal Hospital permission to euthanize my dog/cat. To my knowledge, it has not bitten anyone in the last 10 days.

Owner's Name: _____

Owner's Signature:_____

Animal's Name:_____

Description: _____

Staff Member's Initials:_____

---

hospital when possible to sign the form. Someone's signature (veterinarian or technician) should appear on the form, acknowledging that the client verbally granted permission for euthanasia. From a legal standpoint, the date is important and must be recorded.

Other Consent Forms

Consent forms for other procedures, such as for surgery and medical treatment, are not used in all practices. In the hospitals that use them, they should be treated like any other medical record.

Make sure the owner understands everything on the form. Do not permit a minor to sign it. Again, it is not a legally binding contract if signed by a minor.

Health Certificates And
Accredited Veterinarian Records

An accredited veterinarian is a licensed veterinarian who has successfully completed additional instruction and training required by the state and federal governments. Only accredited veterinarians can sign health certificates and forms for interstate transport of animals. If the veterinarian is not accredited, forms for interstate shipment must be sent to a state agency for approval.

State requirements for shipping change often, especially those for large animals. Staff members may be asked to keep these interstate shipping requirements updated by noting any changes in a notebook (Fig 8). If you are handling the mail, never throw out dispatches from state regulatory agencies.

In most practices, health certificates for small animals are issued most commonly. The interstate forms are valid for only 15 days; therefore, the client's visit to the veterinarian

Figure 8. Requirements for interstate shipment of animals can be recorded in a notebook for quick reference. This sheet summarizes requirements for importation of cattle to New York state.

State	ID No	Bruc Class	TB	Bruc	Herd Test	Anaplasmosis	Bluetongue	Cattle Scabies	Vesicular Stomatitis	Prior Permit (518) 457-2886	90-Day Quarantine
Alabama	64	A	X	X	X*	X	X				
Alaska	96	Free	X	X							
Arizona	86	Free/A	X	X	X*	X	X	X	X	X	X
Arkansas	71	B	X	X	X**	X	X	X		X	
California	93	A	X	X	X*	X	X	X			
Colorado	84	A	X	X	X*	X	X	X	X		
Connecticut	16	Free	X	X							
Delaware	50	Free	X	X							
Florida	58	B	X	X	X**	X	X			X	X
Georgia	57	A	X	X	X*	X	X		X		
Hawaii	95	Free	X	X							
Idaho	82	A	X	X	X*	X	X	X			
Illinois	33	A	X	X	X*	X	X	X			
Indiana	32	Free	X	X							
Iowa	42	A	X	X	X*			X			
Kansas	48	A	X	X	X*	X	X	X			
Kentucky	61	A	X	X	X*	X	X				
Louisiana	72	B	X	X	X**	X	X			X	X
Maine	11	Free	X	X							
Maryland	51	Free	X	X							
Massachusetts	14	Free	X	X							
Michigan	34	Free	X	X							
Minnesota	41	Free	X	X				X			
Mississippi	65	B	X	X	X**	X	X			X	X
Missouri	43	A	X	X	X*	X	X	X			
Montana	81	Free	X	X		X	X				
Nebraska	47	A	X	X	X*	X	X	X			
Nevada	88	A	X	X	X*	X	X				
New Hampshire	12	Free	X	X							
New Jersey	22	Free	X	X							
New Mexico	85	A	X	X	X*	X	X	X	X		
North Carolina	55	Free	X	X		X	X				
North Dakota	45	Free	X	X				X			
Ohio	31	Free	X	X							

should correspond to this time frame. The patient must be examined by the veterinarian issuing the form because the veterinarian must certify the animal is free of skin lesions and infectious diseases. The form is supplied by the Department of Agriculture in the state of origin. Figure 9 illustrates an unofficial health certificate. Figure 10 shows the official form for interstate or international shipment of animals from New York state.

Figure 9. Unofficial health certificate.

Health Certificate

This certifies that on this _____ day of _____, 19_____, I have examined the following described dog _____ cat _____ breed _____ sex _____ animal's name _____ age _____ color _____ property of: _____ _____ address _____ _____ and, to the best of my knowledge, I have found this animal to be free from infectious or contagious diseases, including rabies.

This further certifies that this animal received _____ (brand of rabies vaccine), Serial No. _____ on _____, 19_____.

Dr. _____

_____

_____

During the visit for a health certificate, the animal should be examined, the rectal temperature recorded, and the dates of recent vaccinations reviewed. Especially important is the date of the last rabies vaccination. For export to Canada, rabies vaccination must be within the previous year. Proof of vaccination, in addition to the health certificate, is neces-

Figure 10. Official form for interstate or international shipment of animals from New York state.

STATE OF NEW YORK - DEPARTMENT OF AGRICULTURE AND MARKETS
DIVISION OF ANIMAL INDUSTRY

INTERSTATE/INTERNATIONAL HEALTH CERTIFICATE FOR DOGS, CATS, POULTRY, ETC.
(Not to be used for bovines or equines)

Use only when the animals meet the import regulations of the State of destination.

Mail all three copies to State Division of Animal Industry, Albany, NY 12235
OR
For International Endorsement mail to:
USDA-APHIS-VS, 5 Washington Square, Albany, NY 12205
Pink copy will be returned to shipper.

Owner	Consigned To
Address	Destination Address
Social Security No. * Federal ID No. *	
Reason for Not Supplying Your SS# and Fed. ID#(See instructions on back of form)*	Shipped by: __Air __Express __Auto(check one)

SPECIES (Dogs, Cats, Poultry, Etc.)	AGE	SEX	BREED - Description	VACCINATION GIVEN Product _____ Type _____ Rabies Other	DATE OF VACCINATIONS

The above described animals were vaccinated as listed above and were found clinically free from symptoms of any contagious, infectious, or communicable disease.

N.Y.S. Vet. I.D. #_____

_____
Signature of Veterinarian issuing chart

Date_____

_____
Printed Name of Veterinarian

_____
Director, Division of Animal Industry

_____
Address

_____Date

_____
Approved

_____
Phone

Approval of this certificate indicates our belief in the honesty and competency of the veterinarian signing same and is not a guarantee of health.

sary for travel (Fig 11). These forms must be available for inspection during travel.

Health certification requirements for large animals vary a great deal, depending on the species. All require that the veterinarian examine and properly identify the individual animal(s) by ear tag, tattoo or drawing.

Frequently, the requirements include blood testing. Tests that may be necessary for large animals include tuberculosis and brucellosis testing in cattle and Coggins' testing in horses. Certain vaccinations may be required before interstate shipping. Time intervals between testing and shipping or vaccination and shipping may be critical. Scheduling for such visits and tests may be the job of hospital staff. Know where to find the information and how to interpret it.

If the staff member cannot specifically answer a client's questions on interstate shipment, the question *must* be referred to the veterinarian. Accuracy in meeting regulations is essential.

Figure 11. Rabies vaccination certificate.

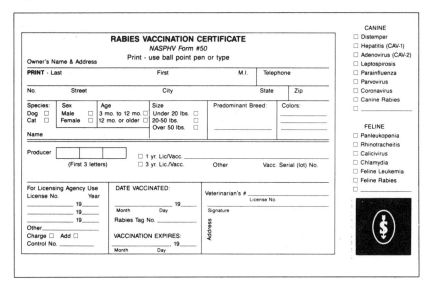

Remember that all signatures on health certificates and forms must be the veterinarian's own. Never sign the veterinarian's name.

Prescription Forms

In human medicine, prescription writing is routine, whereas it is much less common for veterinarians to write prescriptions. Veterinarians usually stock most of the drugs they use on their animal patients. Nonetheless, hospital staff should be aware that a need for a prescription might arise. If the hospital does not stock prescription forms, a prescription can be written on office stationery.

A prescription must include the veterinarian's name, address and telephone number. Some states also require the veterinarian's licensure number and the BNDD/DEA registration number. The client's name and address, patient's name and species, and the date should also be recorded on the form. The veterinarian fills out the prescribing information (drug name, dosage form, quantity to dispense, dosage interval, instructions for administration) and signs the form.

Medication Labels

Veterinary technicians often fill out medication labels according to the instructions of the veterinarian. Frequently, the orders are oral or handwritten abbreviated notes that the technician must understand and be able to accurately transcribe into comprehensible directions for the client.

Read the instructions to the client, watching for signs of confusion. Ask the client if the instructions are clear. Do not use abbreviations or shorthand on medication labels because you may be the only person to understand or remember the shorthand.

Tamperproof and childproof vials are recommended by most states and agencies. In some states they are required and have replaced envelopes. Labels should include warnings, such as "poison if ingested," "wash your hands after using" or "give after meals." Many of these warnings are available in sticker form for affixing to vials.

A listing of the local Poison Control Centers should be easily available to staff members in case of accident. Also, an updated, alphabetized collection of package drug inserts can be very valuable. If the hospital does not have such a file, this would be an important contribution that a veterinary technician could make.

Submission of Rabies Specimens

Hospital personnel are often required to fill out paperwork and forms for rabies sample submission to a state diagnostic laboratory. In many states, rabies specimens are packaged in special containers, which are available from the local health department. Several containers should be obtained for later use. The sample submission form requires information on species of animal, date when signs appeared, date of death and, if applicable, owner, method of euthanasia, immunization and the name of anyone who was bitten or exposed.

In most cases the veterinarian prepares the rabies specimen and provides the containers and forms. It is the responsibility of the client to submit the specimen and bear the expense of testing (if any). You may be the person who must explain this in such a way as to guarantee no misunderstanding.

The best method for shipping rabies specimens is to have the client take them in person by automobile to the laboratory doing the testing. The next best way is to ship by

United Parcel Service (UPS). If the client is concerned that people have been exposed to their possibly rabid animal, the sample should be transported by the client. The client most often will wait at the hospital until the specimen is readied and then transports it to the laboratory or the UPS office. You must be prepared to issue directions to the UPS office and the laboratory. In some communities, the Board of Health assumes the responsibility for transport of rabies specimens.

The veterinarian prepares the specimen. For large animals, the brain or brainstem is removed, while bats and similar small mammals are sent whole, with the head intact. Methods of euthanasia should not involve destruction of brain tissue. If you are advising a client who wants to dispatch a fox from the family's porch and test it for rabies, tell the client not to damage the head, as from gunshot.

Other Specimen Submissions

All test forms should be filled out completely and accurately. Tissue specimens and slides should be packed securely. The form should include a complete history, as well as the stains or fixatives used, and the times and places of collection. Samples for certain clinical chemistry assays, such as blood ammonia concentrations, require very specific handling and packaging to ensure accurate results. A veterinary technician must be aware of these special requirements.

For Review and Discussion

1. Who owns an animal's radiographs?

2. You are given the job of creating additional room for animal medical records in the existing files. How would you do this?

3. What are the differences between the chronologic and problem-oriented formats used in animal medical records?

Recommended Reading

Nelson AW, in McCurnin D: *Clinical Textbook For Veterinary Technicians.* 2nd ed. Saunders, Philadelphia, 1990.

Pratt PW: *Laboratory Procedures for Veterinary Technicians.* 2nd ed. American Veterinary Publications, Goleta, CA, 1992.

Rumore JJ *et al:* Medical records and the law. *JAVMA* 178:202-205, 1981.

Notes

Chapter 5

Notes

6

Inventory Control and Ordering

An inventory of controlled substance drugs is required by law by government agencies. In addition, an inventory should be a requirement for good veterinary hospital management. An inventory of all drugs and supplies provides information on which drugs and supplies are physically available for use and which items are on order. It also aids in the development of reorder points and purchasing.

A hospital staff member is often given the responsibility, wholly or partially, of maintaining the drug inventory and a list of manufacturers or distributors, with their addresses, telephone numbers and sales representatives. Included in drug inventory duties can be receiving, unpacking, listing and pricing drugs and supplies. Finally, the responsibility for returning expired or defective drugs or supplies may also be part of the duties. The next most logical step in hospital management is to involve the same person in ordering.

The cost of drugs and supplies comprises a significant percentage of a veterinary hospital's expenses. Drugs and supplies are necessary to properly conduct business. Suppliers expect to be paid for these goods within 30 days of billing. Maintaining an adequate but minimal inventory is good hospital management and increases the business profit.

Inventory control may appear at first to be complex and difficult to deal with. However, if each individual area is studied and understood, the composite picture will be clear.

Legal Aspects

In a veterinary hospital the responsibility for establishing medication use and dispensing rests with the veterinarian(s). Staff members must be cognizant of the laws regulating the use and dispensing of drugs so that they do not unwittingly break the law or place the veterinarian's license in jeopardy.

Controlled Substances

The Controlled Substances Act of 1970 classified certain drugs according to human abuse potential and established dispensing limits, distribution restrictions and necessary inventory and use records. The Act is enforced by the Drug Enforcement Administration (DEA). The drugs of concern are categorized as Schedule I, II, III, IV or V, with Schedule-I drugs having the greatest potential for human abuse and dependence. Schedule-V drugs have the least potential. Schedule-I drugs are used for research only.

Veterinarians using these drugs must obtain a DEA license number. To obtain Schedule-II drugs, such as morphine and barbiturates, a special federal written order form must be used (Fig 3 in Chapter 5). Purchase records for Schedule-II to -V drugs must be kept for a minimum of 5 years. A log of use of these drugs (used in-house or dispensed) must also be kept for 5 years (Fig 2 in Chapter 5). Schedule-II drugs must be logged separately from all other scheduled substances. An initial inventory of controlled substances must be taken and followup inventories done every 2 years.

The law states that controlled substances must be kept locked in a double-locked safe or cabinet (*eg*, a locked metal box containing the drugs kept within a floor safe or locked wall cabinet).

State Pharmacy Laws

There are state laws regarding controlled substances as well. Local DEA offices or individual State Boards of Pharmacy can provide state law requirements.

Most states require that dispensing records be easily retrievable. Their concern is the possibility of accidental human ingestion of drugs dispensed to animals. Of prime importance is the name of the drug and the amount of drug dispensed.

State laws also govern labeling requirements. The hospital's name, address and phone number, client's name, patient's name and species, date, veterinarian and directions for drug use are the usual state requirements. Because state laws vary, it is best to check with each state. Auxiliary labels may also be required. Examples of these "stick-ons" are "Poison – External Use Only" and "Shake Well Before Using."

Federal Drug Laws

The Food, Drug and Cosmetic Act of 1938 requires that the consuming public be provided with drugs that are safe and effective. The Durham-Humphrey Amendment in 1951 classified drugs as prescription or nonprescription. Prescription or legend drugs are available only through licensed veterinarians and other licensed health professionals. These drugs bear the legend "Caution! Federal law restricts this drug to use by or on the order of a licensed veterinarian" or "Caution! Federal law prohibits dispensing without a prescription."

Staff members should never refill or dispense medications without the veterinarian's approval. This is especially important when dealing with prescription drugs. Though nonprescription drugs can be sold directly to clients, labels stating the warnings as well as instructions for proper use must be affixed to containers of these drugs. To distinguish prescription from nonprescription drugs, look at the legend.

The Poison Prevention Act of 1970 requires that oral human medication be dispensed in childproof containers. This law does not apply to veterinarians. However, most state veterinary societies suggest the use of childproof containers for animal medication.

Inventory Control

Staff Responsibility

Inventory control should be the responsibility of one hospital staff member. Ideally, this same person should also be responsible for drug ordering. In this way, only one inventory system is used and only one person must be consulted when questions or problems arise. Expired drugs, double ordering and forgotten orders are less likely. The same person doing inventory and ordering should also receive and unpack the goods as they arrive at the veterinary hospital.

Responsibility for inventory control is important, but it is not a duty that is performed on a daily basis. In most hospitals, the workload is greatest during the first and last weeks of the month. Time to concentrate on this portion of the job must be granted to allow the proper discharge of duty and to minimize errors.

Location of
Drugs and Supplies

There are only a few alternatives in locating the pharmacy within a veterinary hospital. One arrangement is to have a complete pharmacy in each examination room. However, the required storage of extra drugs would require a larger examining room, and though time might be saved in dispensing drugs for every office visit, inventory control and pharmacy management would become increasingly difficult with each additional examination room that is stocked.

Having a single central pharmacy in the hospital makes inventory control more manageable. The labor required for record keeping, inventory and ordering is reduced. However, the drawback of a central pharmacy is that the labor and time spent with each office visit are increased because the technician or veterinarian must walk to the central pharmacy to obtain the needed drugs.

The most common arrangement is a combination of these 2 approaches. A limited quantity of commonly used supplies and drugs is stocked in each examination room, while a central pharmacy is used for storage and dispensing of most goods. Examples of items in the examination rooms include syringes, needles, cotton, bandaging and routinely used injectables. This provides an efficient method of treating common problems while minimizing clutter. A record can be kept of supplies and drugs taken from central pharmacy storage to stock examination rooms; in this way inventory control can be managed from the central pharmacy.

Drug Arrangement in a Central Pharmacy

There are many possibilities for arranging drugs and supplies. The system employed in a hospital is often arrived at after some trial and error. Few systems are so structured that they cannot be altered or modified as the situation dictates. Often a veterinary hospital employs a combination of the ideas suggested below.

In all cases, drugs and supplies must be stored on shelves and counters somewhere in a room. The most practical storage system uses the room so that shelving is on 3 sides; this allows both visual and manual contact with all the supplies and drugs from the center of the room. Refrigeration should be available in the central pharmacy to store biologics. Some hospitals also have small refrigerators in each examination room.

The shelving should be adjustable to handle various sizes of containers and numbers of units purchased. Common storage items include gallon containers, flea spray, cotton rolls and ointment tubes. For the convenience of staff members, the shelving must be arranged for people who are between 5'2" and 6'4" in height. Similarly, counter height and depth should be determined according to who uses the counters and for what purpose.

Alphabetic Arrangement: Drugs and supplies can be arranged alphabetically from A to Z (from acepromazine to cotton to zolazepam). This very simplified method is easy to arrange.

Classification System: Drugs and supplies can be classified by their use. Examples of classifications include antibiotics, antidiarrheals and anthelmintics. Such supplies as syringes, cotton and gauze would be in a supply section.

Categoric Arrangement: Another arrangement for supplies is by category. Under this system, capsules and tablets are located in one section, injectable pharmaceuticals in another, biologics, gallons, ointments, narcotics and surgical supplies in other areas. This system is easily managed and understood, and handily used by staff members.

Numeric System: A less common method is a strict numeric system. Each drug and supply item is issued a number and then stored accordingly. A list of the numbers with the corresponding items is available in the pharmacy. Though seemingly a simple arrangement, much time and effort can be expended checking the list to find the location of a given drug.

Most veterinary hospitals employ a combination of these systems. The laboratory, radiology and surgery areas may have their own supply storage areas. Gallon containers and ointment containers may be stored alphabetically, and all other drugs may be stored by classification, such as antibiotics, etc.

The simplest and most familiar method for the hospital is the best method to use. However, if problems continually arise during inventory control and ordering using a certain pharmacy arrangement, a change in system might be warranted.

Storage Restrictions

Drugs and supplies must be stored according to their storage restrictions. Read the label and package insert for storage precautions. Assume that all drugs are unstable and will deteriorate if improperly stored.

There may be adjectives rather than temperatures used to describe storage conditions. If adjectives are used, such as cool or warm, you must be able to associate a temperature with them. The following definitions are from the U.S. Pharmacopeial Convention.

- Ideal refrigerator temperature (36-46 F)
- Ideal freezer temperature (-4 F)
- Cold environment (not exceeding 46 F)
- Cool environment (46-59 F) (These products can be stored in a refrigerator unless the label warns against it.)
- Room temperature (59-86 F)
- Warm environment (86-104 F)
- Excessive heat (above 104 F)
- Protect from freezing (Freezing can result in a loss of product potency.)
- Nonspecific storage conditions (If there are no stated limitations, the item should be stored to protect it from moisture, freezing and excessive heat.)

A thermometer should be used periodically to check refrigerators, freezers and storage rooms to make sure the appliances are operating properly and the storage room is within the temperature guidelines. The main concern with storage is protection from freezing and excessive heat. To be certain that drugs are stored at the required temperature, a list should be developed for each storage requirement and the drugs listed under each.

Monitoring Current Inventory

The inventory provides information on what is in stock. In addition, it provides information pertaining to the quantities of items used by the hospital over a given period and the cost of each item. These data are valuable when drugs and supplies are ordered or when quantity buying is contemplated.

Inventory counts in a veterinary hospital should be conducted at least once a year. In most hospitals, inventory is done much more often. Knowledge of current inventory is necessary for ordering and, because orders are generated monthly, inventory is usually done at the same time.

Some hospitals use a computer program to simplify inventory control. Items received are entered into the program and, as prescriptions are written, drugs and supplies are methodically removed from the inventory. At any given time, a printout can be produced, listing the drug and supply in stock. Expiration dates, costs and manufacturers are also easily obtained from such printouts.

When a computer is not available for inventory control, manual methods are used. Information on each item or drug is maintained in a ledger or on an inventory card (Fig 1). Pertinent data include the drug name or item, supplier,

Figure 1. A sample inventory card.

Inventory Date ___/___/___

Item: _____

Size/Concentration/Type: _____

Expiration Date:_____

Suppliers:_____

_____

Cost Per Unit: _____

Quantity in Stock: _____

Reorder When Quantity Below: _____

Economic Order Quantity (see page 76)

    Quantity in stock, date_____

    Quantity ordered, company, date _____

    Quantity received, date _____

expiration dates, cost per unit, quantity bought, quantity on hand, and date of the current inventory count.

Ordering Supplies

Turnover

Drugs and supplies are ordered, arrive at the hospital and are unpacked. They are placed in storage, used and eventually reordered. The time between the arrival of the drug and reordering of that same drug is called the *turnover rate.* It is measured in days and is a very important time to calculate.

Though hospital policies vary, the ideal turnover time for each drug should be between 30 and 45 days. Using the 30- to 45-day ideal turnover time, drugs on hand longer than 45 days are classified as *low-turnover items,* while those used in less than 30 days are classified as *high-turnover items.*

At first glance it would seem beneficial to manage inventory so as to have all items classified as high turnover. However, if items must be reordered in less than 30 days, this low-volume purchasing system often does not allow one to take advantage of occasional discounted prices. Also, purchasing drugs in less than 30 days increases the actual cost of drugs. Time involved in reordering, transportation costs, and lost opportunity for delayed billing offset any apparent gain with drugs used in less than 30 days.

Drugs held for more than 45 days are also a problem. This situation indicates a miscalculation and too large a purchase of slow-moving items. This occurs most commonly with seasonal items, such as heartworm preventive medicine and flea control products. Previous seasonal use numbers may not pertain to the current year, resulting in low turnover.

Overstocking also occurs when a drug is ordered because certain doctors have used it in the past. Circumstances change, veterinarians make substitutions, clients move and patients die, resulting in low turnover of certain drugs. Use past records, common sense and intuition in ordering. Set a goal of 30-45 days as the turnover rate for each item.

Reorder Point

A well-managed pharmacy has drugs and supplies available when they are needed. Often there is no alternative drug that can be substituted if the required drug is out of stock. To avoid this possibility, the veterinary technician must establish a *reorder point* for each drug and supply in the hospital. The reorder point is the minimum amount of the drug or supply allowed in the hospital inventory. When that point is reached, the item must be reordered to avoid a shortfall.

To establish a reorder point, you must determine the rate at which the item is used in the hospital. The record of use is shown by the inventory card, computer program or a supplier's printout. By checking the interval between previous orders and the number of units ordered each time, you can calculate the average number of units used each day.

Another necessary determination is the time required to obtain another supply from the distributor, including the number of working days for shipment. Normally, if an order is placed by telephone before 10 AM, the drugs are shipped the same day. Biologics are an exception to this rule. Because these items must be refrigerated, distributors may not ship if there is any possibility of a weekend delay. Biologics are therefore best ordered early in the work week (Monday, Tuesday).

Knowing the drug use rate and the required shipping time, you can establish a reorder rate. Following is an example for 250-mg tetracycline capsules:

- Use rate: 25 capsules/day
- Shipping time: 4 days
- The reorder point is therefore 25 x 4 = 100 capsules.

When the inventory of 250-mg tetracycline capsules falls to 100, that drug must be reordered to prevent a shortage. The reorder point should be established for each drug and recorded on the inventory card.

Order Quantity

The next calculation is the quantity to order, so as to ensure that the turnover rate on the drug is 30-45 days. In the example above, tetracycline is sold in quantities of 100, 500 and 1000 capsules. Knowing all the facts, an order of 1000 capsules is best (25 capsules/day x 30 to 45 days = 750 to 1125 capsules needed).

Want List

Every hospital has a place for staff members to record a request for a drug or to indicate a potential drug shortage. This is often called a *want list*. Any staff member who sees a potential shortage is encouraged to use the want list.

In addition to a want list, the person in charge of inventory periodically determines which drugs and supplies are needed. Using inventory records and reorder points, the necessary quantity of drugs and supplies is determined. The order is then placed by mail, FAX or, most likely, by telephone using the supplier's toll-free 800 number. The drug supplier is often a distributor. Distributors sell the products of many drug companies and also sell their own generic brands. Some manufacturers do not sell through distributors; therefore, if the hospital wants their products, an order must be placed directly with that manufacturer.

Drug companies and distributors send sales representatives to veterinary hospitals on a routine schedule. Their visits are usually 4-6 weeks apart. At each sales call, the sales representative will gladly accept an order for drugs and supplies. Many are also willing to check the hospital's inventory and do the ordering based on that inspection. Few veterinary hospitals avail themselves of this service, however.

If drug orders are placed by telephone, obtain the name of the person taking the order. If problems develop, having the name of a contact person at the company involved can simplify resolution of the problem.

The veterinarian should be consulted before ordering a drug in a different dosage form, color, quantity or package (*eg,* a capsule instead of a tablet).

An example is a tablet that is prescribed for cats to maintain acidic urine. When you buy these tablets from Company A, they are colored red. The same drug is available from Company B at a lower price, saving the hospital 1 cent per tablet. These tablets from Company B are colored blue. Many clients refill prescriptions for this drug on a monthly basis. Though staff members can tell clients that the blue pill is the same as the red pill, many owners may not believe this and may later attribute any inefficacy or problems to the "new drug."

Timing an Order

To avoid a shortage, you must be prepared to place an order when the reorder point is reached. The ideal ordering time is on or shortly after the 27th of the month. The supplier expects payment for an order by the 10th day of the month following the date of the invoice. Many companies allow an additional 1-2% discount on bills paid by the 10th. If a bill is not paid on that date, most companies add a 2% finance charge.

Example:

- $1,000 due Ajax Company by June 10th.
- If paid by June 10th, discount 2%, pay only $980
- If paid after June 10th, add 2%, pay $1,020

The key phrase is "by the 10th day of the month following the date of the invoice." By ordering at the end of the month (the 27th or later), the invoice is prepared in a new month and payment is actually due 2 calendar months away. The invoice is usually prepared and sent a few days after the drugs are ordered.

Example A: Ordered May 27th, invoiced June 1, balance due July 10

Example B: Ordered on May 24th, invoiced May 28, balance due June 10

In example A, the hospital that ordered on the 27th would have the drugs to use and dispense for an additional 30 days before payment is due. If the hospital is operating on a 30- to 45-day turnover rate, the inventory will be near zero and the purchased drugs will have generated the income to cover their cost by July 10th. In example B, the earlier payment date (June 10) does not allow sufficient time to generate capital to pay the bill.

Business people, including veterinarians, should be concerned about cash flow (dollars generated by the business as cash, excluding accounts receivable) compared with the dollars owed by the business. There is a decided advantage in having a positive cash flow, *ie,* more money coming in than is owed. If the veterinary hospital is operating as a predominantly cash business, purchasing as many drugs and supplies near the end of the month and maintaining a 30- to 45-day turnover rate enhances cash flow. The drugs are received and sold. This cash can then be used to pay for those drugs.

The Economics of Buying and Selling

Determining An Item's Total Cost

The *total cost* of an item (TC) is more than its *invoice cost* (IC) because it also includes the *ordering cost* (OC), the *inventory* or *carrying cost* (CC) and the sales tax.

An item's *total cost* (TC) can be calculated as: TC = IC + OC + CC + tax. The invoice cost is the cost of the item, per unit, as charged by the supplier. For example, the heartworm preventive for dogs, Heartgard-30 (disc of 6 tablets, 10 discs to the box) costs $76 a box. You order 1 box. The $76, or $7.60 per disc, is only the invoice cost.

An item's *ordering cost* (OC) is a hidden cost but a cost, nevertheless. Consider everything that must go into an order: checking the inventory, selecting the drug, researching the best price, placing the order, and then receiving it, coding and eventually paying for the order. For example, the OC of Heartgard is estimated to be $5 per box; therefore, in this example, $5 is added to the cost of the box, or 50 cents per disc. The total cost is now at $81 per box or $8.10 per disc.

The inventory or *carrying cost* (CC) must also be considered. Several items are factored into this cost. First is overhead expense; each square foot of the veterinary hospital costs money to build, maintain and staff. There is insurance required for the building and its contents, including inventory. In the example, Heartgard has an expiration date of June, 1995. If not sold and used by then, the drug must be replaced. Instead of buying the drug, the hospital could have placed the $76 in a savings bank and drawn interest on it. This is called the alternative opportunity cost. Again, someone calculated these carrying costs at 25% of the purchase price. In our example then, the hospital must add $19 per box or $1.90 per disc as a CC.

The final cost consideration is taxes. The hospital must pay a sales tax on most items. A 6% tax adds $4.56 to the box and 46 cents per disc. At this point the true total cost can be calculated: TC = IC + OC + CC + tax.

- Per box @ $76 (IC) + $5 (OC) + $19 (CC) + $4.56 (tax) = $104.56

- Per disc $7.60 (IC) + $ .50 (OC) + $1.90 (CC) + $.46 (tax) = $10.46

In determining the selling price of an item, all the costs must be considered to avoid incurring a loss. What appears to be a high profit for the hospital on each item sold is not necessarily so. Proper pharmacy management entails constant checking and updating of original drug costs and taking advantage of specials and volume buying.

Economic Order Quantity or What Is the Best Deal?

Sales representatives estimate that technicians order the drugs in over 50% of veterinary practices. Giving technicians this responsibility is a trend that has been increasing for several years and continues to escalate. Veterinary technicians and other staff members are commonly involved in both the ordering of drugs and in decisions regarding volume buying.

Meeting the Turnover Rate: Drug companies and distributors frequently offer special deals, giving large price breaks with volume purchasing. Initially, these appear to be opportunities to save money on drug costs. However, consider carefully before accepting any apparent bargain.

When a deal is offered, check the inventory to see if there is a need for that drug, especially in the volume suggested in the transaction. Certainly, if there is a need and the turnover rate of 30-45 days can be met, the purchase becomes an excellent one.

Expiration Dates: Unless the turnover rate can be met, beware of short-dated items. These are drugs and supplies whose expiration date is in the very near future. Know each company's policy on expired goods because some companies will replace expired goods or credit your account, while others will not. Of course, if the expected turnover rate is favorable, short-dated items may be a good purchase.

Storage Requirements: A year's supply of some items, such as containers of flea spray, can require a great deal of storage space. It may be possible to agree to a volume purchase, thereby saving dollars, but have the shipment delivered over a year's time, thereby reducing the storage requirement and spreading out the payment process. Divided shipping allows you to take advantage of the volume price break while maintaining the expected turnover rate.

Example: Eighteen gross of flea spray are offered for an excellent price. Eighteen gross are used in the practice over 1 year, mostly from June to November. You arrange for 6 deliveries of 3 gross each to be sent on the 28th of each month starting in May. Storage requirements are reduced, the turnover rate is approached, the timing of the order meets cash flow needs, and a lower unit price is guaranteed.

Customer Preference: Sales of some items are based on customer preference, such as mastitis formula, pet vitamins and shampoo. If the consumer changes product preference, you can be left with a large volume of such items.

Even after considering all these factors, it may be difficult to decide whether to take advantage of a special offer. A mathematical formula has been devised to determine the most economical volume for a purchase, known as the *economic order quantity* (EOQ). The derivation of the formula is as follows.

The ordering cost (OC) has been established at $5 per item for each time the item is ordered. If an item is ordered 10 times a year, the ordering cost for the year on that item is $50. If, however, the hospital only orders it once a year, the OC is $5. Therefore, the fewer times the item is ordered, the lower the OC.

Conversely, the greater the quantity of purchased items, the greater the carrying cost (CC). The CC is 25% of the invoice cost. Therefore, $100 worth of a drug has a CC of $25, but $1000 worth of the drug has a CC of $250.

The total cost (TC) of a drug is the invoice cost (IC) plus ordering cost (OC) plus carrying cost (CC) plus tax (TC = IC + OC + CC + tax). Because the tax is a set amount, a constant, the important variables in the total drug cost are the IC, OC and CC. Purchasing in quantity lowers the unit price of a drug but increases the total IC.

Example:

- Regular purchase: 1 box = $76 IC
- Volume purchase: buying 36 boxes reduces unit cost to $70.
- IC = 36 × $70 = $2,520

Mathematically, the point where the total cost is the lowest is where the decreasing OC meets the increasing CC. That point has been designated as the *economic order quantity* (EOQ). The EOQ is the most economical quantity to order of a particular drug or supply item. The EOQ can be established for every ordered item or for only the more commonly used or expensive items. The inventory card shown in Figure 1 contains space for the EOQ. The EOQ can be used to determine if a special offer is a good deal.

$$EOQ = \sqrt{\frac{2\ (OC)+(AD)}{CC}}$$

AD = units ordered in a year; $\sqrt{\ }$ = square root.

Using the Heartgard example, the hospital's *annual* need (as determined by the inventory) is 20 boxes. Our OC is $5 and the CC (25% of $76) is $19 per box.

$$EOQ = \sqrt{\frac{(2\times5)+(20)}{19}} = \sqrt{\frac{200}{19}}$$

$$= \sqrt{10.5} = 3.24, \text{ rounded off to 3}$$

Computations are easily done on pocket calculators. The EOQ = 3 units, meaning that the most economical ordering quantity for Heartgard is 3 boxes.

Example: The drug company offers the hospital the following deal: Purchase 10 boxes of Heartgard at one time and the price per box drops to $70. Should you take advantage of this deal? Use the total cost formula, TC = IC + OC + CC. If the hospital's annual purchase is 20 boxes per year, what is the total cost of buying 1 unit at a time as compared with 3 units at $76? Further, what is the total cost of 10 boxes at $70 per box?

By comparing these figures you can see:

- At \$76/unit, the most economic quantity to order is 3 units.

- If a price break is offered and the quantity (10) does not exceed the annual demand (20), this particular deal would be advantageous to the hospital.

Cost/Unit Purchases	\$76/Unit 1 Unit	\$70/Unit 10 Units
(IC) 20 units/year	\$1,520	\$1,400
(OC) \$5/unit/order	100	10
(CC) 25% of unit cost x units	19	175
Total Cost	\$1,639	\$1,585

Determining an Item's Selling Price

The selling price of an item is typically determined by doubling the purchase price and adding a fixed cost. The fixed cost is added because of several factors, including the veterinarian's time to prescribe the drug, the technician's time to fill the prescription, the cost of the drug vial, and the receptionist's time to find the medical record, record the transaction and replace the medical record. If the purchase is charged, there is an additional cost to the hospital. The fixed cost figure is a constant whether the prescription involves 10 capsules or 100 capsules.

For example, if the hospital's policy is to double the purchase price and add a fixed cost of \$1 per prescription, what should a client be charged for 1 disc of Heartgard?

- IC = \$7.60 + 6% tax = \$8.06
- Double the IC = \$16.12
- Add the fixed cost of \$1 = \$17.12

• Round up to nearest quarter = $17.25

The hospital's total cost of a disc, adding IC, OC, CC and tax, is $10.46. Therefore, the hospital's profit for each disc sold is $6.79.

Prepackaged and Repackaged Items

Prepackaged items include shampoos, anthelmintics and ointments for eyes, ears and skin. They are convenient, they carry labels and warnings, and they are timesavers in a busy practice.

Many of these items can be purchased in multi-unit containers. For example, shampoos are frequently purchased in gallon jugs rather than 4-ounce containers. They can be repackaged from the large containers to more practical sizes for dispensing. Repackaging would seem to produce a large profit; however, one needs to calculate the time needed to repackage, losses from spills and breakage, and the additional costs of labels and warning requirements. When all these factors are determined, repackaging of most items is not economically practical.

Receiving Shipments

As previously mentioned, it is good hospital management to assign to the same staff member who orders supplies the duty of receiving and unpacking them. If this cannot be arranged, only one person should be involved with receiving, unpacking, marking and cataloguing incoming items. If more individuals are involved, no one remembers what was delivered and efficiency is reduced.

Packing Slip

Items are usually delivered by United Parcel Service (UPS), US Postal Service or truck carrier. The goods are boxed with a packing slip attached to the outside of one box or enclosed within a box. The *packing slip* lists what the shipper believes has been sent. You should locate the packing slip and make sure it is correct.

Unpack the shipment carefully, and itemize and compare the contents with those listed on the packing slip. Note the quantity and size of each item. A thorough search through the packing material may be needed to locate small items. Then the drug and supply order list should be compared with the packing list to confirm that all ordered goods were sent and received.

Returning Items to a Supplier

The company should be contacted immediately if there is a problem with a shipment. If possible, talk with the person that recorded your order. Have the packing slip available so that you can supply the order number and the packer's initials.

Never discard any item without permission from the shipper. If the wrong item, number or size was shipped, the company may want it returned by carrier or may send a sales representative to pick it up.

Damaged Packages

You can refuse to accept delivery of severely damaged packages. Depending on the contents, you may be able to ascertain the extent of damage without opening the package. For example, liquid contents soaking a box certainly is not normal. Do not sign for damaged goods delivered by UPS; have the driver return the box. Items delivered by the Postal Service can be taken back unopened to the Post Office for return. Call the supplier immediately. When possible, retain the original packing slip and return a copy to the shipper.

Usually a package that appears damaged must be opened and inspected. If the goods are damaged, notify the shipper immediately, thereby putting them on notice that ordered items did not arrive in satisfactory condition. Request replacements for the damaged items to avoid shortage in the pharmacy.

Bookkeeping

Many hospitals have a bookkeeper who writes the checks to pay for drugs and supplies. The bookkeeper must be informed of all shipments. Packing slips, once checked for accuracy, are given to the bookkeeper. If there is a problem with an order, a paper trail is initiated so the bookkeeper can properly handle payments. Notes and memos should be complete and accurate.

Biologics

Biologics (vaccines, bacterins) are usually shipped under refrigeration to avoid deterioration of the product. If they arrive either warm or frozen, alert the supplier and seek replacements. Warm biologics are not acceptable.

Recording Receipt of Shipments

Each drug or supply item must be recorded on receipt. This may be in a log, on an inventory card or perhaps on a computer program. Important information to include is the date the drug was received, quantity, size, dosage form and price. The drug should be placed in the pharmacy in the appropriate area. If current inventory is still available, rotate the drugs so they will be dispensed according to expiration dates (older drugs dispensed before newer drugs). Expired drugs must be removed from inventory.

Expired Goods

There is great variability in company policies on handling expired goods. Some companies give credit on goods returned before the expiration date, others give credit only after the drugs are outdated, and some do not give any credit on expired drugs. Companies may have you destroy expired goods or may require that they be shipped back for credit. They may ask that the goods be retained by the hospital until a sales representative arrives to verify and accept the drugs in question. Learn each company's policy for expired goods.

Back Orders

Back orders are an annoying but common problem. When a supplier does not have an item that was ordered, their inventory has become depleted so they cannot fill your request. You may be told this at the time of placing an order or discover it when examining the packing slip.

The supplier may fill your back order on a given day, or the delivery date may be unknown. You must now make a decision. Based on current inventory, it may be possible to wait for the back order to arrive; however, if waiting is not practical, you must search for other distributors or manufacturers for replacement. Before canceling the back order with Company A, make sure the drug is available from Company B.

A log or list should be kept of all back-ordered drugs and supplies, including the company and the date of back order. As back-ordered items arrive, they are removed from the log. The bookkeeper should be kept current on the situation.

Occasionally a back-ordered drug may be removed from the market. If this happens, inform the veterinarian so that a substitute can be selected.

Interaction With
Sales Representatives

Sales representatives, like drugs and supplies, come in a variety of packages. Their incomes depend largely on volume of products sold. The better their service and line of merchandise, the more the hospital will buy.

Services provided by sales representatives include supplying information about special deals and new drugs, handling damaged and outdated goods, and correcting shipping errors. Many sales representatives now have computer printouts of a hospital's drug orders. These printouts can be helpful in determining seasonal needs and previous use figures. Sales representatives should also describe the company's shipping and return policies. Some companies offer free shipping with quantity purchases.

"Detailing" new drugs is an important function of sales representatives. This is an in-depth explanation of a drug's actions, benefits, uses and potential in a veterinary hospital. The drug's advantages are often illustrated with brochures and perhaps even videos and films. Reviewing this information is time consuming. Most veterinarians do not wish to spend time with every sales representative; therefore, the staff member responsible for ordering often does the listening for the veterinarian.

Always be courteous to sales representatives. Establish certain days and especially times of the day when you are free to talk with them. Inform them of these times and be prepared to visit with them then. Representatives must visit 10 or more hospitals in a day and do not desire a long wait in the reception area.

Your responsibility is to pass along information on new drugs to the veterinarian. Procure the drug data, add notes, highlight portions of a brochure with a marker and document pricing. The veterinarian will need the data to decide whether to purchase a new item.

Some sales representatives are personal friends of the doctors. Find out which representatives the veterinarian wishes to speak with personally and coordinate the meeting. A few pleasant minutes with an old friend and catching up with the local gossip may be an enjoyable respite for a practitioner.

For Review and Discussion

1. While unpacking drugs at your hospital, you read the following statements on the drug labels: Avoid excessive heat. Keep frozen. Store at room temperature. Must be kept refrigerated. Protect from freezing. At what temperatures would you store each drug?

2. Your hospital uses 250-mg amoxicillin capsules at the rate of 15 capsules per day. Shipping time is 2 days. What is the reorder point for this drug?

3. Your hospital works on a 30- to 40-day turnover. Amoxicillin is sold in quantities of 100, 500 and 1,000 capsules. Which amount would you order?

Recommended Reading

Lane D: Taking charge of your inventory. *Vet Economics* 29(8):42, 1988.

Notes

7

Employee
Supervision

The majority of a veterinarian's time is spent treating sick animals. This is what they want to do and have been trained for. Doctors are happy to delegate a portion of the hospital's management to interested and competent members of the veterinary staff. Reasons for a staff member to take on administrative duties include the personal satisfaction of excelling in many areas of the profession and the opportunity to move forward in a career with increased responsibility, salary and prestige.

Staff members who can work and deal with people are candidates for management of service promotion and employee supervision. Personnel managers are faced with many challenges, such as hiring proper employees, solving personnel problems and even firing of employees.

Skills Needed
For the Job

Employee supervisors must have good verbal and writing communication skills. Verbal skills include the ability to talk sensibly and easily, not only with other technicians and lay employees, but also with veterinarians and clients. Equally important is the ability to listen and to assimilate and understand their input.

Writing skills are required for producing recruitment brochures, job descriptions, employee schedules and recommendations. Correct grammar, spelling and accuracy are necessary basic skills. Typing ability or basic computer or word-processing knowledge may be necessary in many employee supervisory positions.

A personnel manager must be a problem solver. Each day's work brings new problems to the job. The personnel manager must represent both the owner and the employees, between whom there may be an invisible barrier. To be effective, a supervisor must be fair, respected by fellow employees and able to solve problems in a swift and equitable manner. Equally important is the ability to recognize possible trouble and remedy the situation before a problem develops. Employee problems often originate with the worker. If a supervisor can envision the needs and wants of a work group and then hire accordingly, many problems never develop.

Employee Needs
and Wants

Employee needs, in the most general terms, include compensation, recognition and social interaction. Compensation includes salary and fringe benefits. Every effort should be made to provide fair and just compensation.

Low salary is a major cause of turnover. A 9- to 15-month turnover of new employees is average, and each turnover is estimated to cost the hospital $500 to $2,500. A supervisor who hires at a competitive salary and provides salary reviews on a regularly scheduled basis will be able to reduce staff turnover. Turnover cannot be totally eliminated, but any reduction is a savings of time and dollars. Moreover, if an employee cannot survive on their salary, that person is dissatisfied. Unhappy workers do not communicate well with clients and other staff members, and they often have a negative attitude that affects everyone.

Employees also have a need for recognition. Supervisors have the opportunity to provide both praise and criticism. Supervisors should always praise their employees in public, especially to a veterinarian or a client. Nothing you can do, short of salary increases, will improve the attitude and efficiency of an employee like praise does. Conversely, criticism should always be in private. Criticism offered in front of peers, supervisors or clients is a bitter pill to swallow. Moreover, criticism should always be administered as constructive suggestions.

Staff interaction is another important employee need. Employees need to feel that they are an integral part of the practice, that their contribution is important and that the hospital's success depends on a team effort. This feeling can be enhanced by positive interaction among the veterinarian, the supervisor and the staff.

A good employee supervisor must be certain that all staff members are aware of changes and the reasons for them. Informal, constructive staff meetings can bring problems into focus so that all can become involved in problem solving. When staff members are uninformed, however unintentionally, they feel isolated, compartmentalized and unwanted.

Long-term employment should be a goal of all employee supervisors. Understanding employee needs and supplying both psychological and monetary compensation result in a happy, long-term association for staff and hospital.

Employer Needs and Wants

A good employee supervisor understands the veterinarian's needs and wants, and hires people who fulfill them. Veterinarians need hospital employees who are both motivated and dedicated. Employees can be taught both technical and nontechnical skills, but motivation and dedication are innate qualities. Employees must be reliable and, above all, good with clients.

Any hint of negativism in a prospective employee should alert the supervisor to trouble, especially before hiring. A negative attitude is infectious and pervasive, and undermines any business, especially one so allied with client relations, such as a veterinary practice.

A common question is whether employer needs or employee needs should be met first. The supervisor must first satisfy the employer's needs and wants. Select the person with the qualifications the employer is seeking, then attempt to meet the new employee's needs and wants.

Hiring the Right People

Advance Preparation

Hiring the right person for a position requires knowledge of each area of responsibility within the hospital. The supervisor must know the skills and personality required for the position. The supervisor may possibly have even worked in that position.

A written job description should be prepared, detailing the responsibilities of the position and the duties required to meet the employer's needs. The written job description is used in recruitment, interviewing, training and supervision. Any special job conditions, such as shift work or weekend hours, must be documented. Any special skills, such as radiographic positioning or anesthesia monitoring, must be noted in the job description. Evaluate and update job descriptions as necessary.

The supervisor must also establish a list of questions to be asked at the interview. The same questions can and should be asked of all candidates interviewed for a particular job. Indeed, many questions may be standard for every position in the veterinary hospital. The candidate's educational background, work experience and career goals should be noted. Ask probing questions and evaluate the candidate's ability to solve problems, handle stress and communicate.

Certain questions cannot lawfully be asked in an interview, including questions on race, marital status, sexual preference, national origin and religion. However, questions on disability, arrest history and citizenship are allowed and may have a bearing on a candidate's suitability for a position. In general, questions must be nondiscriminatory and lawful. Sample questions are found in Figure 1.

Where to Find Candidates

There are a variety of places to look for prospective employees. Some are better than others and all have limitations. Knowing the position and the necessary qualifications, select a combination of advertisements that will best reach the candidate you want. The following discussion uses an example of a veterinary technician position. A basic requirement is a licensed or license-eligible technician; experience is desirable.

The pool of candidates can come from a variety of sources. Many applicants write, call or appear in person at the hospital. They may be local residents or recent graduates looking to relocate. Instructions should be given to all staff members on how the supervisor wishes job applicants to be processed. There may be an opening in the near future even if there is no current opening. Potentially, each candidate could be a fine employee; applicants should not be dismissed because of the way in which they applied. Try to draw from the largest possible group of qualified people.

Classified ads in the local newspaper, specifically stating the qualifications and salary range, are another source of applicants. Hiring veterinary technicians by this route is often difficult. People may not read or may refuse to believe your stated qualifications. The result can be a flood of applicants, none of whom meets your needs. Conversely, the ad could produce exactly what you want. The best approach may be to list a post office box where inquiries and resumes should be sent. This allows you to make your selection without identifying your hospital.

The supervisor can target the market by advertising the position in trade papers or journals, such as state veterinary newsletters, the *Journal of the American Veterinary Medical Aassociation (JAVMA)* and manufacturers' publications. A disadvantage of these publications is that it may be months before an ad appears. Moreover, though veterinarians see these publications, veterinary technicians may not.

State veterinary technician societies may have newsletters or publications. Though the time lag remains a factor, you can be sure that veterinary technicians will see the ad. *Veterinary Technician,* published monthly by Veterinary

Figure 1. Examples of questions asked during interviews of veterinary staff candidates. These questions are slanted toward veterinary technicians.

- Why did you choose _____ College?
- Are your college grades an indication of your true abilities? Why?
- What courses in college will help you the most in this job?
- What campus organizations or activities did you participate in?
- Did you participate in off-campus groups and activities? Which?
- What past work experiences will help you most at our hospital?
- Describe your last job and your responsibilities.
- Can you get positive recommendations from your previous employers?
- What did you especially dislike about your last job?
- Do you prefer working with others or by yourself? Why?
- How do you feel about overtime work?
- Have you held leadership roles at work or in organizations?
- How do you rate yourself as a supervisor?
- What personal characteristics are necessary for success as a veterinary technician?
- What do you see yourself doing 5 years from today?
- What are your strengths?
- What are your weaknesses?
- What books have you read recently for enjoyment?
- Who is your favorite author?
- Why have you decided to go into practice?
- Why have you decided to relocate to (city)?
- Why would you like to work at our hospital?
- What are your salary needs?
- What 2 accomplishments have given you the greatest satisfaction?
- Why should we hire you?

Learning Systems, has a large circulation and can be used for advertising.

Write to schools in your state or area of the country that have technician programs. Remember to include your alma mater, even if you have moved out of state. Program directors at each school can often locate candidates for you. In addition, directors often hear about graduates who are contemplating a change. Many colleges also provide a placement service that includes a bulletin sent to their graduates. This type of advertisement gets your message to the experienced veterinary technician.

Before the Interview

Selection starts with an evaluation of the resume. The supervisor should review its format and appearance. Have some thought and organization gone into its preparation? Are the grammar and spelling correct? Does the applicant fulfill your requirements for education and experience? If the answer to any of these 3 questions is "no," then this candidate may not be suitable for the position. Compare the resumes of all the candidates and then rank them. This forces you to critically survey the candidates.

Screen this initial list by evaluating several criteria. Review the candidate's recent jobs for length of service. Compare employment record with the time frame. Are there significant periods of unemployment? Are there patterns to the work experience? Make notations of any questions so that you can clarify them in an interview. Often there are valid reasons for termination of employment; the candidate should be given an opportunity to explain the circumstances.

Some hospitals have formal application forms for candidates screened to this point. Application forms vary in both length and in detail. An application can request more information than a resume provides; for example, personal history (name, address and telephone number, and position desired). Questions concerning citizenship, felony convictions, physical limitations can be asked. Questions about previous employment would include the names, addresses, supervisors, dates of employment and reasons for leaving. Usually 3 references are requested, none of whom should be relatives. Their names, addresses, telephone numbers and relationship to the applicant are important. Included in the application should be a request for permission to contact both present and past employers.

Supplemental data sheets may be part of an application. These request the candidate's name, place of birth, birth date, sex, race or ethnic group, veteran status and handicaps or disabilities. These data sheets state that the applicant's submission of this information is voluntary, and that the hospital will not use it in consideration for employment. This information is submitted to the government in periodic reports as required for Equal Opportunity/Affirmative Action Employers.

Interviewing

Meet candidates in a quiet, comfortable area free of distractions, such as intrusions and telephone calls. Be punctual, dressed professionally and well groomed. Attempt to place the candidate at ease. Judge the candidate's answers with consideration to organization, thought and common sense. Watch for answers that could tell you something about willingness to work, motivation and degree of sincerity. Use a prepared question list so that all candidates are asked similar or the same questions (Fig 1). Evaluate candidates in terms of grooming, dress, language and grammar, in addition to qualifications.

Provide the prepared job description to thoroughly acquaint the candidate with the position and its duties. Encourage questions from the candidate and evaluate the quality of those questions. Does the candidate appear truly interested in employment at this hospital? Are his or her questions concerned with understanding the job, the duties and the responsibilities, or is the candidate more interested in salary, vacation time and other fringe benefits?

Salary and fringe benefits should be discussed at this or future interviews. Be sure that you have accurate information concerning these areas and know the salary limits.

The interview is terminated with a job offer, a rejection or a delayed decision. Be sure to state the reasons for your course of action. Usually the decision on hiring is delayed. If you require time to conduct additional interviews, be sure the candidate understands when a decision will be made. Followup contact is necessary. Always thank the applicant for their time.

Contact the references if the candidate is otherwise acceptable. A telephone contact is quick and easy, and allows more frank appraisals of the candidate than written contacts. Your perceptions of the candidate should be comparable with those of the reference. There may be areas where the applicant is weak. If these areas are not critical to the position and can be developed and improved, they can be overlooked.

Employees of the hospital who have had contact with the candidate may be consulted for their opinion of the candidate. Personality quirks, likes and dislikes may have been revealed during these sessions. Each new meeting involves a first impression; the supervisor has one and each employee involved also has one.

Job Description

Proper hiring takes a great deal of time and energy. You must be thorough and convinced that the employee hired is the best one available.

Once a candidate has been offered the job, the duties, wages and fringe benefits must be explained very clearly and recorded in the form of a written agreement. When the candidate accepts your job offer, a starting date is determined. If the candidate requests time to consider the job offer, be sure the time allotment will not jeopardize filling the position if this candidate turns down your offer.

The new employee's first day should include a review of the job description and a presentation of this written description to the employee. A personal orientation should follow, with introductions to all staff members. Hospital policies should be reviewed and given, in written form, to the new employee.

Training New Employees

The employee supervisor is the person who reviews personnel and hospital policy, and answers new employees' questions. Areas to cover include the dress code, vacation days, sick leave, fringe benefits, time cards, paydays, job description and training period policy. The new employee should initial a dated copy of the hospital's personnel policies.

Dress Code

A hospital dress code is a method of achieving a professional look and staff conformity. Because of the expense involved, most hospitals with a dress code reimburse the staff with a uniform allowance. An explanation must be given of how the allowance may be used, the amount and the necessary documentation.

Personal Leave

Employees accumulate vacation time, sick days and personal days. The new employee must be given the hospital's definitions of these days, as well as the policy for requesting leave. The regulations should be straightforward and clear.

Fringe Benefits

Fringe benefits offered to employees at a veterinary hospital may include health insurance, continuing education allowances and technician association dues. Hospital personnel often have pets, and there may be a hospital policy for treatment of employees' animals.

Time Cards

Large hospitals often use time cards or another method of signing in and out of the work day. The new employee should be told how to sign in for work each day. Certainly, a discussion of paydays and method of payment is appropriate.

Job Description

The job description should also be reviewed again. This written document describes the duties of the position, thereby informing the new employee of the hospital's expectations regarding job performance. The duties should be described in detail so that there is no question regarding what must be done and whose responsibility it is to do it.

Training Period

A formal training period for new employees is a good management tool. The written job description can be used as an outline. The new employee should be trained by the supervisor or a designated employee. Sufficient time for training varies with each position. Safety instruction should be included in the training. For veterinary hospitals, safety includes the animal patient's safety, as well as the employee's safety.

After an appropriate training period, the new employee's performance should be evaluated by the supervisor. Additional training may be necessary. A new employee is not fully trained until the supervisor is satisfied with the employee's progress and performance at assigned duties. A new employee should expect review sessions with the supervisor.

The job description is used in evaluation of an employee; therefore, in addition to a listing of responsibilities and detailed duties, a good job description should also establish acceptable performance standards and the consequences of inadequate performance. A detailed job description is preferable to a flexible document, with which neither the employee nor the supervisor has a full understanding of the obligations and authority involved.

Scheduling Work Hours

Scheduling of work hours is usually assigned to the employee supervisor. Work days are scheduled so that sufficient help is always available, especially during peak periods or days. Understaffing causes anxiety and stress for employees, while overstaffing can result in boredom.

A successful schedule plans for normal occurrences, not the exceptions. A supervisor cannot plan for emergencies that extend the day or poor weather that can cause cancellations. A rule of thumb is to have 1.5 to 2 technicians per veterinarian on duty.

Because of the long hospital work day, staff coverage must be overlapped. Arrival and departure times for staff should be staggered by 30 minutes so that adequate coverage is ensured. Lunch periods must also be staggered.

Overtime should be avoided. An abundance of overtime can make employers unhappy. A good supervisor must strike a happy balance in arranging staffing coverage.

Example:

- Work day runs from 8:00 am to 6:00 pm
- Office hours are 10 am to noon and 1 pm to 6 pm
- Veterinarian A works 8 am to noon and 2 pm to 6 pm
- Veterinarian B works 9 am to noon and 1 pm to 6 pm
- Veterinary technician A works from 8 am to 5 pm, with a lunch break from noon to 1 pm
- Veterinary technician B works from 9 am to 6 pm, with a lunch break from noon to 1 pm
- Veterinary technician C works from 9 am to 6 pm, with a lunch break from 1 pm to 2 pm

With this schedule, surgery and office hours are covered. Employees have a lunch period, and the office is always staffed. There are 1.5 veterinary technicians per veterinarian with this schedule.

Ideally, the schedule and the work days should be varied. This allows staff members to eventually work with all other employees, and develops greater flexibility and diversity. Employees also have an opportunity to improve in various areas of the practice. Continued attempts by the supervisor to rotate schedules and staff reap several benefits: staff members develop improved skills, animal care is better, working conditions can be more equitable, and the entire hospital operation becomes more efficient.

Personality conflicts and employee desires to work with certain people or in certain specialities can create scheduling problems. Acknowledge employee likes and dislikes but attempt to maintain a harmonious work atmosphere; however, do not schedule personnel according to their personal life style or preference. Covering the hospital's needs must be the first consideration; if possible, individual desires can be factored in.

Handling Personnel Problems

Personnel problems constantly arise, and a good manager must be able to solve them with minimal disruption in the workplace. A supervisor must make every attempt to be fair. Each person views both the problem and the solution in a different way, and no one is always right or always wrong.

A supervisor must be assertive and firm, always maintaining control of the situation. If an employee suspects indecision on the part of a supervisor, control is lost and the solution, at least in the employee's mind, is not satisfactory. Being firm, fair and consistent in making decisions can be difficult for managers. Decisions can be even more difficult if the supervisor socializes with employees. When a situation involves a friend, other employees will question whether the supervisor's solution is fair and consistent. Unfortunately, therefore, social contacts with employees must be minimized if you are to be an effective manager.

To make the correct decision in a personnel problem, you must obtain all the relevant facts. The details must be weighed, sifted and balanced. Be sure that you have considered all aspects of the problem, but do not allow too much time to elapse in attempting to make a perfect decision. A "perfect" judgment may be arrived at too late to be of any value.

When you make a decision, personally inform the parties involved. In this manner, the resolution is public, rumor is eliminated and the participants have a chance to question you directly. Follow through on any difficulties to be sure that the decision is binding.

If you find that a particular decision turns out to be incorrect or counterproductive, amend the decision in whatever way is necessary to correct it. An error is difficult to admit, but a faulty decision is harder yet to live with. A good manager will acknowledge a poor decision and remedy the mistake.

Performance Reviews

Regular performance reviews should be scheduled at the time of hiring each employee and this schedule should be followed. Employees should expect to be evaluated by the supervisor on a regular basis. These evaluations are the only way to officially inform employees of their progress. Conduct employee evaluations in private. Relate positive feedback on performance before you make any critical comments.

The written job description is a useful instrument in a review. This is an excellent opportunity to modify the job description if necessary. Discuss mutual problems with the employee and attempt to resolve them. If a problem is not amenable to a quick or easy settlement, the supervisor must set a deadline for a resolution. The discussion should also establish attainable goals for the employee. These goals include short-range objectives to meet before the next performance review, in addition to long-range goals.

The supervisor should follow the verbal discussion with a written evaluation. The written form should include an overall evaluation based on the job description. If the duties have been changed or modified, this also should be noted. Mutual problems should be stated, as well as decisions or pending dates of resolution; established goals should be specified.

If the employee's performance is rated as substandard, both employee and supervisor should agree to terms for improvement. Establish a period within which the employee's performance must meet the job standard. Another review should be scheduled at the end of that period.

The supervisor should also be prepared to reward exceptional performance by an employee. Kind words are the minimum reward; greater motivation is gained with monetary reward. If a wage increase is impossible, explain this to the employee.

Stress Management

An employee may not meet work obligations because of a poor understanding of the position, lack of ability or stress. A poor understanding of job duties can be corrected with a review of the job description and extra training. Improved screening can prevent hiring an employee who lacks ability. The work problems created by stress may be more difficult to ascertain, prevent or correct.

Signs of stress in an employee include reduced work quality, increased errors and absenteeism. Absenteeism is easily verified by checking the employee's records. Compare attendance over specific periods to see if there is a correlation with the reduced work quality. Discussions with co-workers and the employee may reveal other signs. People who are stressed often have difficulty making decisions and then they agonize over those decisions once they make them. Stressed employees may have outbursts of temper, or they may become forgetful. The presence of some or all of these signs may convince the manager that stress is a real problem.

Stress may be related to on-the-job problems or personal problems. Personal problems may involve health, finances or interpersonal relationships. Though aid and support can be offered for off-the-job situations, the supervisor will find that solving on-the-job problems is easier.

The supervisor can make several suggestions to employees to help them cope with stress. Suggest that the employee work at being positive about everything. If certain coworkers have a tendency to be negative, help the stressed employee to avoid those coworkers. Make a daily list of tasks to complete; avoid too long or demanding a list. Completing all the tasks before leaving gives an employee a sense of accomplishment.

If the problem is job related, temporarily change the employee's duties to work in another area with different staff members. Ideally the new situation should be one where the everyday problems are different and the atmosphere is more relaxed. Having something new to look forward to is helpful in combating on-the-job stress.

Dismissals

The personnel manager must know how to dismiss an employee when necessary. Formal performance evaluations are important in this process. A verbal warning can be given initially to the employee with a substandard informal evaluation. Establish a time limit for improvement. If unsatisfactory work continues, a warning must be given in writing. Make a written report of all formal evaluations. Written documentation of poor performance or unsatisfactory conduct should be standard procedure for a supervisor. There can be legal repercussions from dismissal of an employee without written documentation.

In certain circumstances, written warnings before dismissal are not necessary. Employees who are insubordinate to the supervisor or employer are subject to immediate dismissal, as are employees who arrive at work drunk, who drink on the job, or who are involved with illicit drugs. Employees who steal from the hospital are also dismissed without a second chance; such individuals violate the trust given to them upon their employment. The wrong message is conveyed to other employees if they are not summarily discharged.

For Review and Discussion

1. What skills are needed to be a good employee supervisor?

2. As a supervisor, you must know employee and employer needs. List the needs of each.

3. What are some possible signs of job-related stress?

Recommended Reading

Fudin C: Enhancing client relations. *Vet Technician* 7:30-31, 1986.

Fudin C: Nonverbal behavior of the human animal. *Vet Technician* 10:319-324, 1989.

Shouse D: How to hire the right people. *Vet Economics* 29(9):58-60, 1988.

Notes

8

Use of Computers

In veterinary hospitals, computers are used most often to maintain financial and inventory records. Other frequent computer uses include communication and storage of financial and medical records.

An increasing number of veterinary clients own and are familiar with computers. Effective computer use in the hospital enhances the practice's image as efficient and modern.

Veterinary staff must become familiar with computers and how to input and retrieve data. The computer is still an underused tool in veterinary hospital management. Staff members who are expert in its use are great assets to the practice.

A detailed discussion of computers is beyond the scope of this chapter, but following is an outline of ways in which computers can be used in a veterinary practice.

Computer Uses In a
Veterinary Hospital

Financial Management

Veterinarians and business managers use the computer
to assist practice management. Programs are available that
generate daily, monthly and annual income data. Important
information on the source of income is available. This income
analysis helps identify financial trends and workloads
within the practice. Expenses can be recorded so that
monthly profit-and-loss statements and year-end balance
sheets can be produced.

In addition, computer programs are used for client billing.
Each charge is itemized, resulting in more accuracy and
fewer client complaints. The computer is programmed by
code; each code is associated with a set fee. Therefore, the
computer takes any indecision out of pricing a service or a
product.

The hospital's payroll data can be programmed into a
computer. A computerized payroll is a labor-saving tool for
the hospital.

Such program data as hourly rates and hours worked are
easily modified with a decided advantage over hand
calculations.

Inventory Control

Computers are used in inventory control. The system
could inform the hospital when to order a product and from
which company. The program can monitor expiration dates
and provide information on heavily used products each
month. Reorder amounts and reorder times can be established so that the computer can generate reorder lists. With
proper data entry, items can be consistently priced. Use of

inventory records allows the hospital to buy wisely when volume buying is offered by drug companies.

Word Processing

Word processing with the computer is an important part of management. Newsletters, hospital forms and brochures can be produced and individualized with a computer. Mailing lists and labels can be generated. A list of medical procedures with current prices can be produced. These documents are easily stored and retrieved and can be changed to reflect current ideas or costs. Multiple copies can be produced, eliminating the cost of using a commercial printer.

Reminder Notices

Client reminders are an important tool in veterinary hospital management. Reminders concerning heartworm medication, vaccinations, fecal examinations and elective surgery are appreciated by the client; they show that the hospital cares and that the client and the patient are important. Clients that return generate income for the hospital. For veterinarians engaged in large animal practice, herd health programs can be set up with a reminder system. The computer can also be programmed to generate memos to the veterinarians and veterinary staff.

Recordkeeping

Recordkeeping is an important function of computers in a veterinary hospital. Information on medical, surgical and radiography cases can be entered into the computer. Lists of patients by diagnosis can be created, and the number of surgical cases by year or by veterinarian can be established. Patient vaccination information and a daily hospital census are additional examples of data that could be made available to the veterinarian.

Handwritten information from the history, physical examination and laboratory tests is recorded in an animal's record by the veterinarian and the veterinary technician. The time involved in typing it into a computer record immediately, or having office staff do it at a later date, may be prohibitive. However, computerizing medical record information facilitates retrieval at a later date.

For Review and Discussion

Discuss the ways in which computers can be used in a veterinary practice.

Recommended Reading

Annual Software Buyer's Guide. *AAHA Trends,* every June/July issue.

Khare M: Managing your money with accounting software. *Vet Economics* 32(5):90, 1991.

Klooz S: Your computer invoice is a marketing tool. *Vet Economics* 33(8):76, 1992.

Lofflin J: What's new on the computer horizon? *Vet Economics* 33(1):67, 1992.

Schroeder K: Computer usage climbs past the halfway mark. *Vet Economics* 32(12):46, 1990.

Notes

9

Client Relations

Today's veterinary hospital staff members must often play several roles. No matter what constitutes your primary job responsibility, you will have some contact with clients. Whether you are a veterinary technician, receptionist or hospital manager, client interaction may be the most important aspect of your job.

Expanding the hospital's client base or increasing the volume of work can be done in a number of ways. The least expensive and easiest way is to please your current clients. Happy clients will refer others to the hospital. The client you are currently working with is important. A hospital staff member is often less intimidating to the client than the veterinarian, and clients will often be more comfortable with you. Their first hospital contact, in whom they place their initial trust and confidence, is usually not the veterinarian. For this reason, hospital staff members play an increasing role in client relations.

Clients, like all other people, have an innate need for recognition. They want to be accepted and understood. A client wants to be considered as an individual, not as a number or a faceless body. To fill these needs you must be courteous, sincere and interested. The ability to explain and resolve problems is important. Client relations is defined as answering to the client's needs and desires.

Communicating With Clients

Satisfied clients are the product of successful client relations. Satisfaction results when there is adequate and appropriate communication with the client. Good communication involves more than saying the right words and doing the right things. Hospital staff members must listen and watch the client carefully to see if they understand the instructions on medicating or caring for their animal at home. Miscommunication can cause problems for the patient. You must be aware not only of what you say and how you say it but also how it is interpreted.

Only 30% of human communication is verbal. The remaining 70% relates to personal appearance, body language and the physical environment. Personal appearance is the first step toward good communication. People retain only 10% of what is said and listen only 25% of the time. By dressing properly, you can improve listening and retention by clients. Try to dress neatly and be clean and enthusiastic. Speak clearly and properly and be positive in your actions and attitude.

The physical environment is also important to good communication. Distractions within the hospital, such as telephones, other conversations and physical activity, create an atmosphere where listening is impossible. The client is often anxious about their animal, and this limits their ability to comprehend even the most clear directions or explanations. Remove these hindrances to understanding by selecting a quiet, private area to deliver important messages.

Verbal communication consists of more than saying the correct words. When explaining a problem or directions, give the client your full concentration. Watch the client's body language; facial expressions and movement of the hands often portray the client's level of attention, alertness or confusion. An observant person can perceive these changes and adjust the discussion accordingly.

The client craves individual attention, so give it. Show a client you care by sitting and fully explaining the situation in a relaxed and direct manner. Concentrate on making important points. Compliment the client where appropriate and provide encouragement and praise. Ask questions to ascertain understanding. Repetition improves understanding and comprehension. Do not hesitate to emphasize important points.

Professionalism

To develop, maintain, or even repair good client relations requires the hospital staff to act in a professional manner. A professional uses proper language. Slang words such as "yeah" and "nope" are never to be substituted for "yes" or "no." Injection is a better choice of word than shot. Anesthetize is more professional than putting to sleep.

Never become involved in an argument with a client. This does not mean that the client is always correct or that you must always assume they are correct. To have good client relations, the hospital staff cannot argue with clients. If a controversy develops, do not become angry. Excuse yourself to provide both parties with a rest period. Evaluate what point the client is making, and try to understand their reasoning. If you feel you can make another attempt to solve the issue, do it. Otherwise, discuss the situation with the veterinarian and ask for counsel. A different staff member may need to settle the dispute.

Treating a client with respect does not mean that you always agree with the client or that you like the client. But a professional should try to consider and understand the other person's viewpoint. Do not be critical and do not dismiss the client's opinions or feelings. A problem may not be immediately resolvable. Explain the problem as you see it and ask if the client agrees. Explain what you will do or try to do to solve the dilemma. If mutual agreement can be reached, set a time goal for resolution and attempt to meet that objective.

Be cognizant of clients' time. If you must put a calling client on hold, be aware of how long they must wait. If a delay is expected to last longer than 90 seconds, offer to return the call. If appointment hours are full but the patient's needs are real, emphasize that the appointment time is only an approximation and that the doctor will fit them in as expediently as possible. If excessive delays develop, attempt to contact the client to reschedule. A professional should respect the client and the client's time.

Interacting With Clients

Greet people with enthusiasm and animation. Even if the actual words are unsaid, your voice should convey your willingness to help the client and be of service. In 100 AD, a Roman poet, Publicus Syrus, said, "We are interested in people when they are interested in us." By greeting people with enthusiasm, you are showing interest in them.

Smile! A smile says "I like you" or "I am glad to see you!" Smiling is inexpensive and contagious. A hospital visit is often not a cheerful time for an owner; their pet is sick and veterinary care is going to cost them time and money. A sincere smile from the hospital staff can change the client's attitude.

Review the medical card before greeting the owner and patient and remember their names. Most people like to hear their name and the patient's name used in conversation. The patient also will respond favorably to a familiar sound. Remembering a name is easier if you relate it to the owner's features or actions. It may often help to write the name several times. When the client calls and says, "This is Mrs. Smith calling back," and you reply, "Boozer is doing great, Mrs. Smith," you create good client relations.

Unless you are close personal friends or have been instructed to use their first name, address each person as Mr., Mrs. or Miss. If a client has a title, such as Doctor, always use it when addressing him or her. This is a matter of respect; the title holder has earned it and usually expects to be properly addressed. Always refer to the veterinarian as "Doctor." In a private setting the veterinarian may request that the title be dropped; however, you should always use it around clients.

Not all conversations with clients deal with clinical matters. Display a genuine interest in the client, with no ulterior motives. For example, if a client mentions to you that she has a son in the army, you could make a note of that on the file card. The next time the client comes in, a review of the file card refreshes your memory, and you might bring up a question concerning the son during conversation. Attempt to have these discussions involve the client's interests. You could also determine a client's interests and encourage their discussion. In the veterinary hospital setting, these interests may involve fishing, or showing, training or breeding animals. Clients, like all other people, enjoy talking about their interests. Practice your listening skills and encourage client talk. You have displayed an interest in the client, thereby increasing their confidence, and possibly developing a friendship.

Make the client feel important but do it sincerely. For example, "Your dog has a beautiful coat," or "That is a smart horse," or "You've done a great job training your 4-H calf." You must be sincere and not overdo the compliments. If the compliment is truthful and sincere, be sure to pass it on.

Choosing Your Words

What you say can be interpreted in different ways. A wise person will thoughtfully consider the answer to a question before speaking. Unfortunately, experience is often the only teacher. For example, a client might ask, "Did Sam bark all the time I was gone?" A truthful answer might be, "Well yes, he was noisy."

The next time the client calls you, she might say, "Hello, this is Mrs. Baldwin. I own Sam. He's the one who barks all the time, and no one there can stand him." To prevent this negative association, a better answer to the question might be, "Sam only barks when he sees me, Mrs. Baldwin. For a minute he thinks it's you. He's always so happy to see you; there must be a great relationship between you."

Interaction with clients is inevitable. Therefore, it is best to make the relationship a positive one with a potentially rewarding future. The result often depends on your actions and words.

For Review and Discussion

1. What factors are important to good communication with a client?

2. You must obtain a history and do a physical examination on a patient. How would you greet the client in the examination room? Be specific.

Recommended Reading

Antelyes J: Taking the static out of client/staff relationships. *Vet Economics* 33(2):64, 1992.

Becker M: Making peace with unhappy clients. *Vet Economics* 33(8):60, 1992.

Catanzaro T: Client encounters of the best kind. *Vet Economics* 31(5):64, 1990.

Immler M: A friendly smile makes a world of difference. *Vet Economics* 32(9):22, 1991.

Remillard J: Handling client complaints. *DVM Management* 23(8):1-4, 1992.

Notes

Notes

10

Telephone Etiquette

Success in veterinary practice depends on a favorable combination of many factors. The foundation for success is based on the ability of the hospital or clinic to attract and maintain a clientele.

The client's first impressions of a hospital operation are important. These first impressions are shaped by hospital staff speaking to potential clients on the telephone. All members of the hospital staff must answer the telephone at one time or another. In some practices receptionists routinely answer most calls. In other practices, veterinary technicians answer selected calls.

Telephone answering is an important part of veterinary clinical management. The first 30 seconds of a telephone call often determine if a lasting relationship with the client will develop. Staff members certainly wish the practice to thrive, so they should take pride in doing an excellent job on the telephone.

119

Answering the
Telephone

The telephone call initiates the image-building process for a client. The person answering the telephone can be either an asset or a liability to the business. If you are unprepared and unprofessional, the caller questions the hospital staff's abilities without ever entering the hospital doors. Conversely, proper telephone answering is a valuable asset to the practice.

Always attempt to answer the phone between the first and third rings. The time factor is important. A quick answer conveys the image of an efficient, service-oriented hospital. This is an excellent beginning of the relationship with the caller. If for any reason the phone is allowed to ring longer than several rings, apologize to the caller for the delay.

Identify the hospital or clinic and yourself. In this way, you have told callers they have dialed the correct number, and, at the same time, you have personalized the conversation with your name. The use of your first or last name is a matter of individual preference. Some people prefer to use "Jane," others "Miss Roberts." Preface your greeting with a cheerful and positive introduction. For example: "Good morning, Delaware Animal Hospital. This is Jane. How may I help you?"

Be sincere when you speak. The best way to project sincerity is to be yourself. Your voice should be pleasant, warm and cheerful. Speak at a moderate volume. Too soft or too loud a voice is neither easy nor pleasant to listen to. An expressive voice conveys your personality to the caller.

Speak at a moderate rate, but do not use a monotone or be robotic in your speech. You can put more expression in your tone by accenting important words and phrases. This adds emphasis, color and variety to your speech. Try to create a mental image of smiling.

Speak distinctly. Clear pronunciation of words is vital. Do not use slang, abbreviations or technical words. Organize your sentences in a logical manner. If you are disorganized, the true meaning of your message may be lost and the caller may interpret it quite differently from what you intended to convey. Clients will not enjoy speaking to you if they must strain to understand. Poor communication can create monumental problems.

Never treat any call as routine. To the caller, this particular call may be very important. Give the client your undivided attention and concentrate on what he or she is saying. As you answer the telephone in the first 3 rings, you may also be nearing the end of a conversation with a client in the office. Do not laugh or talk to others as you answer the telephone because it is discourteous. Such behavior creates an immediate bad impression for the caller.

Be calm when you talk. You may have another caller on a second telephone line, children in the reception area climbing the furniture, a client who is attempting to talk to you while their dog growls, and a bleeding dog being carried across the parking lot to the front door. Be calm. If you allow the excitement, irritations and distractions of the moment to be carried through your voice, the caller's mental image of a competent hospital staff is destroyed.

Clients may not enjoy the call to a veterinary facility. Inquiring about a hospitalized, injured or ill pet or arranging an office or farm visit can be unpleasant. The caller may be agitated or aggravated, and perhaps distraught and unhappy. Your task is to change the tone of the conversation. Pleasantness is contagious. A positive attitude, a smile and a good word are soon mirrored in people you talk with.

Telephone Manners

Always be courteous on the telephone. Good manners are appreciated by the caller. "Thank you," "please" and "you're welcome" are positive and powerful words that build a good reputation for you and the practice. Some calling clients are angry and discourteous. Do not allow their poor manners to influence your selection of words or your demeanor. Be professional at all times.

Being a good listener may be difficult; however, when answering the telephone, you must be more of a listener than a leader of the conversation. Demonstrate interest and attentiveness by occasionally interjecting such phrases as "I understand, Mr. Jones," or "Yes, sir." Becoming a good listener is a learned trait and a valuable one to develop.

Attempt to be helpful. Clients with a problem require a sympathetic and sincere listener. You are often going to be a problem-solver also. "How can I get my cat to the hospital?" and "I am not able to get Joshua to take the medicine," are examples of problems for which you can find a solution.

Telephone Delays and Transfers

In a busy hospital with a busy telephone, delays are inevitable. There are many reasons why the telephone call cannot be completed immediately to everyone's satisfaction. Apologize to the caller if there is to be a delay in answering or connecting the call.

You may need to transfer a call to someone who has more knowledge of the situation. Transfer the call only when you cannot handle the request yourself, and explain to the caller exactly what you are doing. Stay with the caller until the transfer is completed. To avoid having to transfer many calls, remember hospital policies or, preferably, have them in writing and easily available (see Chapter 1, Standard

Operating Procedures). For example: "A dog that is hospitalized or boarded must be current on the following vaccinations . . . ." or "Full payment of the bill is expected at the time of service unless prior arrangements are made with the veterinarian."

A complete understanding of the hospital routine requires extra work on your part. Each employer's policies and standard operating procedures may be different.

Placing the Caller on Hold

Callers are more likely to be placed on hold if the hospital has more than one incoming line, but placing them on hold is all too common, even with only one line. Being placed on hold is irritating to a busy or anxious client or to a long-distance caller. Piping pleasant music into the telephone is just a happy way of saying, "You're being ignored."

Placing a caller on hold closes that telephone line to any other incoming or outgoing calls. Not only have you created an unhappy caller, you have limited the potential for hospital business by eliminating your telephone service. Therefore, the "holds" should last no longer than 90 seconds. Leaving someone on hold for longer than that is one of the worst telephone offenses.

If you cannot connect the caller to a problem-solver within 30 seconds, explain that the transfer is still pending and ask, "Do you want to keep holding?" If the caller says yes, return again in 30 seconds, apologize for the delay and ask the same question. If the caller continues to hold, return in another 30 seconds and say, "I'm sorry; I'm not able to complete the transfer. May I ask the veterinarian to return your call, or would you prefer to call back?"

In each discussion you have given the caller an option: to wait on hold, to have the call returned or to call back. Also, the telephone line has not been occupied for longer than 90 seconds. Note also the way in which the last question was asked: "May I *ask* the veterinarian to return your call?" The wording is preferable to "I will *have* the veterinarian return your call." The word "have" denotes finality and implies that the return call *will be made.* For any number of reasons the veterinarian may not be able to return the call, thus creating hostility toward the hospital.

If the caller chooses to have the call returned, it is important that every effort be made to return it. The person waiting for the call will be very upset if no one calls them. Clients are lost in this way, however, emergencies do arise that may prevent the veterinarian from calling back, in which case someone, preferably the person who took the message, should contact the caller to explain the delay.

If the client chooses to call back, tell him or her the best time to call. Make sure the veterinarian will be available, or, if that is impossible, attempt to get the question answered so you can complete the inquiry.

There will be times when you need to leave the telephone for information to complete the call, such as to check medical records. This requires 2 hands and undivided attention. Explain to the caller what you intend to do and how long it will take you. Try to complete the call if it can be done quickly, rather than returning the call.

Choosing the Right Words

The person answering the telephone or greeting a client should be tactful and discreet, and use proper terminology. Your choice of words is very important. Consider the following examples.

"Please have a chair in the waiting room." Who wants to wait? A better choice of words would be,

"Please be seated in the reception area." An entirely different and more acceptable concept is conveyed to the client.

"I'll take Henry and put him in a cage." Their dog will now be imprisoned! Instead, "I'll take Henry to the medical ward." Isn't that where he is going and doesn't it sound more professional?

Similarly, your choice of words can create the wrong impression. For example, "The veterinarian is busy; can you call back?" Some clients will think, "I am also busy!" Better ways to say that the veterinarian is unavailable include "The doctor is in surgery" or "The doctor is on a house call" or "The doctor is with a client."

If a caller's request must be denied because of hospital policy, give a straightforward and sympathetic explanation. For example, a typical request might be, "I want to come in and pick up some eye ointment for my dog." However, hospital policy prohibits dispensing of medication over the telephone. "If we may make an appointment for the dog, the examination will determine the best medicine for the eye" is a much better reply than the common answer, "You'll have to come in for an appointment."

Screening Calls

At some hospitals, calls are screened by obtaining the names of the callers. Screening calls is not a recommended telephone procedure because it can irritate clients and make an unfavorable impression.

What is the best method to obtain the name without irritating the client? Callers usually identify themselves withoiut being asked. If not, avoid asking "Who is calling?" This statement is too abrupt and gives the impression that their response to "who is calling" will determine the kind and amount of service they will receive.

A better way to phrase this question would be, "May I tell the doctor who is calling?" or "The doctor is with a patient at the moment. May I take a message and ask her to call you?" You will obtain the same information without causing offense.

Telephone Messages

Be prepared when you answer the telephone. Always assume you will need to take a message. Have paper and pencil or pen immediately available at each telephone. There are a variety of telephone message forms available commercially, or you can develop one of your own (Fig 1).

The date and time of a call are important to the veterinarian who receives the message. Record the caller's name. Try not to interrupt the caller except to gain correct spelling of a name or clarification of a number. If you miss the name or

Figure 1. Sample telephone message form.

Message For:		
Date:	**Time:**	**Taken By:**
Caller:		**Telephone No:** ( )
Address:		
Message:		

cannot spell it, ask the caller to identify themselves again. Proper spelling is imperative in locating records.

An advantage of writing the name early in the conversation is that you can later use it. A mark of a good listener is to use the caller's name in conversation. Do not use the caller's first name unless you are friends. "I understand, Mr. Jones" is an example. There is no sweeter sound to people than their own name. Using their name shows that you have heard the message and you are listening. The only name callers would cherish more than their own is the patient's name. For example, "Mr. Jones, how is Lucky handling this hot weather?"

If the caller wants the call returned, record the appropriate telephone number. This may be a work number or a home number. Both numbers may be necessary, depending on work schedules and time of day. Include the area code if it is different from the hospital's. Repeat the telephone number(s) to be sure they are correct.

Not every caller is a client. Pharmaceutical and equipment sales representatives and other business people may call for the veterinarian. In this case, the firm's name should also be noted on the message.

Be concise in the messages you write. Not everything the caller says must be included on the message form. One way to record a proper message is to write important data on another sheet, using abbreviations if necessary. After the conversation is finished, summarize the most important parts of the message and copy the summary on the message form so that the veterinarian can quickly review it. On the copy, use abbreviations only if the veterinarian can understand them. Keep the original scratch paper for further interpretation or to answer questions.

A pencil is the most practical writing instrument because errors can be erased and corrected. If the message includes a special request, such as "Return call by 4:30 pm," highlight that portion with a marking pen. Highlighting draws attention to important parts of the message. Signing or initialling the message helps the recipient to locate you to obtain additional information or clarification.

Other Considerations

Keep a list of important numbers close to the telephone. The list might include numbers for the local animal shelter, boarding kennels, local pharmacies, animal control agents, wildlife rehabilitators, dog groomers, and poison control centers. Such a list is a time saver and gives a caller the impression of efficiency.

If you are expecting a return call but must be away from the telephone, leave word at the main desk when you will return. Invariably, the return call will come in while you are gone.

If you are busy discharging a patient, for example, when the telephone rings, the best policy, if possible, is to have someone else answer that call. Common courtesy dictates "first come, first served." Give the first client your complete attention until the transaction and conversation are completed.

Using the telephone at work for personal conversations is unprofessional and is looked on unfavorably by your coworkers and your employer.

Making Outside
Telephone Calls

Members of the hospital staff may need to place return calls to clients, drug companies or other businesses. When making a business call, check to see if there is a toll-free 800 telephone number. Using 800 numbers saves money for the hospital. An 800 directory is an excellent resource.

When calling, organize your message and have all the necessary reference material close at hand so you can keep the conversation as brief and business-like as possible. Allow the other party 10 rings (approximately 1 minute) to answer. When calling, consider time zone differences.

If your call may be lengthy, ask whether the other party has time to talk. Always be pleasant and courteous. Obtain the name of the person you speak with. This is especially important when placing drug orders. Later on, a question or problem is much easier to resolve if you have the name of the person you talked to initially.

If a return call is required, give your name, your telephone number and the best time to reach you.

Ending the Telephone Conversation

Use good manners and be courteous when ending a telephone conversation. "Thank you for calling," is preferable to a simple "goodbye." The best policy is to allow the caller to hang up first. They may have an additional thought or comment, and if you hurry to end the call, you might miss the comment, creating a negative image. In all cases, cultivate the habit of replacing the receiver gently.

Traits of a Good Telephone Receptionist

If you become involved in selecting a person to answer the phone, be they a receptionist or a veterinary technician, look for pleasantness, helpfulness, courteousness, friendliness and knowledge.

For Review and Discussion

1. What would you say if you were answering the telephone for the Delaware Animal Hospital?

2. What is meant by "be prepared when you answer the telephone"?

3. If a calling client must be placed on hold, how would you handle the situation?

4. You become an employee supervisor in a veterinary hospital. You must advertise, interview and select a person whose major job description will be to answer the telephone. What traits would you look for?

Recommended Reading

Dooley D: *The Successful Veterinary Receptionist.* (audiotape program). American Veterinary Publications, Goleta, CA, 1985.

Remillard J: How to avoid telephone responses people dislike. *DVM Management* 23(3):1, 1992.

Remillard J: Getting the most with telephone contact with clients. *DVM Management* 22(4):1, 1991.

Swope J: Building your image by telephone. *VM/SAC* 76:1363-1366, 1981.

Notes

11

Client Education

An animal owner who understands the various problems, diseases and conditions that can affect their pet becomes a good client for the hospital. When educated by the hospital staff to be aware of potential problems or situations, the client is more likely to inquire about abnormalities rather than to disregard them as unimportant. Responsible owners understand, through client education, that the prevention of problems is important for the health of their animals.

The entire hospital staff is involved in client education, starting with the owner's first telephone call or visit and continuing at each contact. Client education may be your most important responsibility. The veterinarian is concerned primarily with diagnosis, treatment and surgery and, in today's busy practices, the hospital staff must assume more of the ancillary tasks, including client education.

Occasionally, the client is reluctant to address seemingly minor questions to the veterinarian and is more comfortable talking to a staff member. The busy veterinarian may appear to be unavailable for detailed question-and-answer periods.

Client education requires the veterinary technician and perhaps other staff members to understand the basics of many diseases, conditions, problems, drugs, administration of medicine, restraint, nursing care and therapy, and be able to coherently convey information to a client. Staff members must also be familiar with the hospital standard operating procedures (see Chapter 1).

Though admittedly a very time-consuming endeavor, if done correctly, client education is an excellent investment for the hospital. Clients return to a practice because they have confidence in the veterinarian's ability to diagnose and cure the problem. The confidence the owner has in the veterinarian is established by their perception of the veterinarian's and the hospital staff's skill, caring and ability. The veterinary staff is an extension of the veterinarian because clients often have more contact with staff than with the veterinarian.

Personal Communication and Client Education

The first visit by the owner to the hospital is often the longest. If he or she does not return, the first visit is also the last. Hospital staff (veterinarian included) who rush through this initial contact may easily alienate the client. An overly short office visit can be construed by the owner as only superficial treatment and a lack of caring for the patient. A way to avoid that negative image is to schedule sufficient time with a new patient and be thorough in the examination and history taking.

Certain client education topics could be routinely discussed during initial visits, such as vaccination or parasite control. Careful explanation of animal health information with clients demonstrates thoroughness and caring by a professional staff.

The one-on-one conversation is the most common form of client education. To ascertain understanding, ask the client questions while explaining a condition. Inquiries like "Have I made this clear?" and "Do you have questions?" will give the owner an opportunity to ask for clarification. The client should be encouraged to talk. Through a 2-way dialogue you can determine the client's understanding.

Brochures and Handouts For Client Education

Personal communication is not the only available form of client education. Drug manufacturers, animal food companies and veterinary publishers produce excellent brochures and handouts covering a variety of topics, from animal behavior to specific diseases, parasitism and nutrition. These brochures and handouts are often distributed free or at nominal cost to veterinary hospitals. The material is technically correct and most often well illustrated. These make excellent references to accompany or substitute for personal communication on a topic of interest.

Handouts can also be developed by the hospital. The addition of computer word processing and the increase in veterinary computerization have allowed hospital staff to develop their own handouts and newsletters. However, it is a time-consuming process and the results are not always of the best quality.

Professionally written handouts on medical, surgical and behavior topics for small animals, as well as care of birds and small exotic animals, are available from American Veterinary Publications (Goleta, CA). *Instructions For Veteri-*

nary Clients contains handouts on over 300 medical and surgical conditions in dogs and cats. *Canine and Feline Behavior Problems* contains handouts on 52 behavior topics. *Avian-Exotic Animal Care Guides* contains handouts on care of cage birds, iguanas, snakes, turtles, tortoises, hamsters, guinea pigs, mice, rats and ferrets. All 3 compilations are also available in computer diskette form, allowing customization of each handout with the hospital name and address, as well as the patient's name.

Each client should be given a brochure or handout on some topic at each visit. These provide additional information on topics of interest and reinforce the words of the veterinarian and hospital staff. Placing brochures and handouts in the reception area is not as effective as handing them out individually. Free literature in a reception area is often ignored, or collected and then ignored by clients. Targeting animal owners with specific, relevant printed material is far more effective.

Hospital staff will find it helpful to note the topic of literature that has been distributed to each client. With such a system you can ascertain which topics have been discussed and where emphasis should be placed during each visit. Client education is therefore kept fresh and current, and unnecessary repetition is minimized.

Brochures and handouts should be selected or designed so they are concise and specific to a problem. Clients lose interest and may miss the important points of a lengthy discussion. When giving material to the client, highlighting particular sentences or portions with a marking pen is an excellent teaching tool. The highlighted area focuses attention on important topics.

Audiovisuals For
Client Education

Audiovisuals include film strips, videos and slides. All of these are good sources of client education. Audiovisuals result in good client comprehension. Being able to view and listen concurrently helps to establish an idea. The message should be short (less than 10 minutes long) and accurate.

Commercial companies produce excellent material. A hospital could produce a personalized video with a camcorder. A tour of the hospital, an introduction to the staff and a statement of hospital policies would be an example. This type of video could be part of the initial visit to a veterinary hospital.

With an audiovisual presentation, the owner receives accurate and complete information that is delivered with consistent enthusiasm. Veterinary technicians and other hospital staff can be ill or busy so that material given by personal communication may be skipped or delivered without emotion. Audiovisuals are always on the job. They can even be loaned to owners to watch at their leisure.

The disadvantages of audiovisuals include the need for special equipment, such as slide or movie projectors, television sets and possibly projection screens. Audiovisual equipment is costly and requires storage space.

For an audiovisual to be effective, the equipment must be readily available to all of the staff. Prolonged setup and tear-down times disrupt busy schedules and discourage audiovisual use. A central place for storage and use is important if audiovisuals are to be effective. The staff must know how to use the equipment.

The Hospital Library

Books and periodicals on animals and veterinary medicine are often part of a hospital's library. These items can easily be used in client education. For example, clients may desire more information about their particular breed of animal. Books dealing with popular breeds can be loaned to interested owners.

Using the Microscope For Client Education

All hospitals use microscopes and perform tests that can be very valuable in client education. Ear mites can be demonstrated on a slide viewed under a microscope. The same is true for parasite eggs, heartworm microfilariae, sperm and skin mites.

Taking clients to the microscope and spending a brief time allowing them to view test results is helpful in several ways. Clients then can understand why their cat scratches its ears, as they watch the mites crawling along the slide. They can visualize the danger of heartworms when watching the microfilariae thrashing in a drop of their dog's blood. The importance of proper treatment is more meaningful when many hookworm ova are seen. The technician's discussion of disease problems then has more meaning, and there is greater client interest in the directions for treatment and prevention.

An additional benefit is that owners are introduced to the laboratory area. They look through a microscope but they also see the blood and serum analyzers, the centrifuge and all the test kits. They may be impressed and tell their friends about this experience with veterinary medicine. Clients often share their positive attitudes toward the hospital and staff with friends and family. This is a bonus of client education.

Possible Client Education Topics

The companion animal topics listed below are grouped in several categories. Though most pertain to both cats and dogs, some are more specific to dogs. Staff members involved in client education should be familiar with each topic listed and be prepared to discuss each with the client. Remember the different forms of communication that are available. These include personal communication, handouts, brochures, audiovisuals, books, magazines, periodicals and the microscope.

Parasites	**Infectious Diseases**	**Nutrition**
heartworms	feline respiratory complex	growing animals
roundworms	feline distemper	maintenance diets
tapeworms	feline leukemia virus	working animals
hookworms	feline infectious peritonitis	pregnant animals
whipworms	canine distemper	lactating animals
coccidia	leptospirosis	geriatric patients
mange	hepatitis	obese pets
ear mites	parvovirus	heart patients
ticks	coronavirus	kidney patients
	kennel cough	FUS patients
	rabies	

Reproduction	**Elective Surgeries**	**First Aid**
heat cycles	ovariohysterectomy	first aid kit
signs of heat	castration	bleeding
selecting a sire	ear cropping	poisoning
breeding	tail, dewclaw removal	traumatic injury
pregnancy check		heat stroke
exercise during pregnancy		convulsions
nutrition during pregnancy		
signs of labor		
birthing		
problems during birthing		
problems after birthing		

For Review and Discussion

1. How does a hospital staff member become involved in client education?

2. Client education is accomplished by using several methods. List the different ways you can pass information on to a client.

3. A client's first visit to the hospital is with an 8-week-old puppy. Plan the client education topics you will attempt to cover in this first visit and a second visit within a month.

4. A client's first visit to the hospital is with a 10-week-old kitten. Plan the client education topics you will attempt to cover in the first visit and the second visit within a month.

Recommended Reading

Kuhns E and Erlewein D: *Instructions For Veterinary Clients.* American Veterinary Publications, Goleta, CA, 1991.

Schwartz S: *Instructions For Veterinary Clients: Canine and Feline Behavior Problems.* American Veterinary Publications, Goleta, CA, 1993.

Whitford RE: Building your clinic's image and income. *Vet Technician* 10:302-304, 1989.

Whitford RE: Winning the client on the first visit. *Vet Technician* 10:360-362, 1989.

Woerpel R and Rosskopf W: *Avian-Exotic Animal Care Guides.* American Veterinary Publications, Goleta, CA, 1991.

12

Grief Counseling

C. Barton Ross and J. Baron-Sorensen

The Process of Grieving

The bonds people form with their pets are often as deep as, and sometimes deeper than, the ones they have with other people. Pets make us feel better when we are ill, comfort us when we are lonely, accept us when we have made a mistake, and love us unconditionally.

The bond with a pet can be broken in many ways. The pet may die of natural causes, run away or be stolen, killed accidentally or euthanized. Clients with a deep emotional attachment to their pets can expect to grieve when they lose them.

Elisabeth Kubler-Ross, MD, was the first to outline predictable stages of the process of grief in her book, *On Death and Dying*. Though she wrote about human loss, the stages can be applied to the loss of pets as well.

Loss of a pet elicits a wide range of emotions in your clients that can be associated with certain stages of the grief process. You can play an important role in the client's smooth transition from one stage to another. The grieving process is not a steady, linear ascent from depression to joy. It can be likened to a roller coaster ride, with ups and downs at every turn. At the end of the ride is a place of resolution and acceptance, where the client will be at peace with what went before. The process could be explained as a "2 steps forward, 1 step back" adjustment that occurs in a normal, time-limited progression.

By familiarizing yourself with the characteristics of each stage, you will recognize where your client stands in this process and be able to shape your responses appropriately. These responses can effectively facilitate the smooth transition from one stage to the next in the process of grieving.

Stages of Grief

The stages of grief include denial, bargaining, anger, guilt, sorrow and resolution. These stages frequently occur in this order, but they can occur in other sequences. Some stages may repeat. Guilt is not so much a separate stage as a pervasive entity that crosses all stages and can hinder progress from one to another.

Denial

Denial, the first stage of grief, may be played out during the first 24 hours if the animal's death is sudden or for several days if a terminal illness has been diagnosed. Denying that an event has occurred is a coping mechanism that cushions the mind against the shock it has received. In the case of a missing pet, denial, doubt and guilt may start to set in and pet owners may begin to bargain in an attempt to alter or modify the predictable outcome of the situation they face.

Bargaining

Clients may bargain with God or another higher entity for the life of a pet, or bargain with the pet itself, trying to make it live. They may offer the pet vitamins, tempt it with its favorite foods, and promise never to scold or neglect it again. Bargaining is a way of keeping hope alive and buying time to fully accept the outcome of the situation. When bargaining does not yield the desired results, anger is a natural response.

Anger

When faced with the loss of a treasured pet, clients may become angry with the veterinarian, technician, office staff, family, friends and themselves. The veterinarian who has failed to "save" the pet, or who has made the diagnosis, may be the initial recipient of the wrath. More often, it is the reception staff members who bear the brunt of the anger, either directly or indirectly. Clients may be fearful of alienating the practitioner on whom they have come to rely. If clients are angry with themselves for overlooking clinical signs or waiting too long to seek care, this self-directed anger, once dissipated, will give way to guilt.

Guilt

Guilt is an unproductive, debilitating emotion that often inhibits progress toward resolution of the loss. It is the enemy of healing and closure and, if excessive, may require the attention of a mental health professional. When guilt subsides, it opens the door for sorrow.

Sorrow

Sorrow, or deep sadness, is the core of the grieving process. Though it can be kept at bay during the early stages through the intensity of denial, anger and guilt, sorrow eventually settles in and permeates all aspects of life.

Sorrow is, in fact, a healing emotion. This is the time when tears flow freely. Clients feel relief and release from the pent-up emotions of previous days or weeks. Tears may come at work, in the supermarket, or while driving down the freeway. Clients may report sleep and appetite disturbances at this time. The practitioner might want to remind them soon after a terminal illness is diagnosed that adequate rest and nutrition are important.

With time, sorrow dissipates and everyday tasks begin to dominate awareness. Tears no longer break through into daily activities, but can surface at more convenient times, such as in the evening after work. Clients then feel more in control and are able to see an end to the intense pain that is true sorrow. They now accept the situation realistically. Resolution has begun.

Resolution

In the resolution phase of the grief process, clients realize that the pet is gone, that no amount of wishing will make it different, and that they will survive the loss that previously seemed engulfing. Now they can look at photographs of the pet and smile rather than cry; they can remember walks in the park in the summer instead of anxious trips to the veterinarian; anniversaries and holidays can be recalled with tenderness rather than despair. During this stage of grief, clients may consider sharing life with another pet for the sheer pleasure of having something warm and furry to hug again.

Loneliness

Regardless of how the loss occurs and how well prepared a client is, all clients feel their lives touched by loneliness.

This can occur in the presence of family and friends as well as in the company of remaining pets at home. The client shared a relationship with the departed pet that was special and separate from other relationships. While other pets, family members and friends can provide company and comfort, they cannot fill the space left by the departed pet. Loneliness arises from this space, and the space will fill slowly as the grief process unfolds. Clients may express anger at losing this particular pet while others to whom they are less attached are healthy and well.

An appropriate response from the staff or veterinarian might be, "Even though you have other pets at home, you'll still be lonely for Taffy. While you're healing from this loss, your other pets will still be there to love you."

A Case Study

The following case study depicts the various stages of grief a client may experience. This example will give you an idea of how the stages of grief are manifested and how you may deal with them.

Mrs. Malloy brings in Maggie, her cat, for a yearly examination. While the cat is being examined, Mrs. Malloy remarks on its distended abdomen. The veterinarian feels the area and suggests an ultrasound examination. The examination reveals an abdominal tumor involving several organs.

When Mrs. Malloy telephones the office the next day, the veterinarian delicately shares this sad news with her. In the course of the conversation, she says that she is having a difficult time believing the test results because Maggie appears to be in good health. She asks if it is possible that the results of the ultrasound examination could be wrong.

Mrs. Malloy is *denying* the results of the test. Denial is the first step toward accepting her cat's fate.

The veterinarian continues by telling her what course of action he would like to take in treating Maggie. He explains the options, which range from referring her to an internist for possible treatment, to choosing not to do anything.

Mrs. Malloy is silent. Then she asks, if it really is cancer, could it have been caused by her well water? She states that she has not had it checked recently.

Mrs. Malloy is feeling *guilty*. She is having a difficult time concentrating on what the doctor is saying to her and is instead looking to blame herself for Maggie's illness. She can only focus on what she might have done to prevent it.

The veterinarian tells her that he will call her tomorrow and asks her to think about if she would like a referral to an internist. When he telephones her the next day, she is very tearful. She says that she is wondering if giving Maggie extra vitamins would help her to fight the disease. She begins to cry, then falls silent.

The veterinarian suggests that she go to see Dr. Smythe. He offers to call and set up a consultation appointment for her and Maggie. She agrees.

Shortly after this, Mrs. Malloy receives her bill for the ultrasound examination and calls the front desk to express her outrage at the cost. The receptionist listens patiently but informs her that she must pay the bill. Mrs. Malloy curtly responds that she will and hangs up.

Mrs. Malloy is now feeling *angry*. She may be genuinely upset at the cost of the procedure, but she is also angry that she received this terrible news about her cat from your office. She probably wishes that she had never approved the ultrasound examination so that she would not have discovered the cancer.

Mrs. Malloy and Maggie have been seeing Dr. Smythe for several months now. Dr. Smythe has kept your office abreast of the situation. The treatment bought Maggie a little time, but she has now taken a final turn for the worse. Dr. Smythe recommends euthanasia. Your office agrees to perform the euthanasia in Mrs. Malloy's home.

On the day of the euthanasia, the veterinarian and technician arrive at Mrs. Malloy's home. She is very calm. She takes them to the spot where Maggie always suns herself. She says that this is Maggie's favorite place and that she would like her to die peacefully here. She pets Maggie lovingly. She whispers how much she loves her and what a joy Maggie was in her life.

Mrs. Malloy has come a long way in the process of grieving. She has now *accepted* her loss and is on the way to *resolving* her grief in learning to live without Maggie.

Replacement

The decision to replace a deceased pet with a new one should be left solely to the individuals experiencing the loss. It should not be influenced by the veterinary staff in any way. Some pet owners choose to bond with new pets before their elderly pets die. Others decide that the presence of a new pet in their homes would be stressful for the older pet, and decide to wait. Some clients may never again adopt new pets. Everyone involved must consider the client's needs, as well as the needs of the current pet.

If a client is trying to avoid the experience of loss by finding a replacement for the pet, bonding with the new pet usually does not occur. The new pet is not accepted as a unique being if the owner wants it to be just like the deceased pet. Often these new pets are given away or neglected. Occasionally a client who had taken good care of a previous pet brings in a pet that has been neglected. This client probably has not bonded successfully with the new pet and may need support in deciding whether to keep it or to find a new home for it. The client may not have resolved the loss of the previous pet and may need to see a counselor or support group that deals with pet loss issues.

Assisting Bereaved
Pet Owners

Clients grieve in a variety of ways. Some demonstrate their emotions, while others may show little if any feeling in your presence. Do not assume that clients who do not display emotion are not grieving. They deserve the same support, courtesy and kindness you give to someone who is openly upset.

Try to assess your client's feelings to determine how much support you should provide. When clients show reluctance to accept concerned overtures from you, take a minute to let them know that you care about their well-being. By acknowledging their sadness, you open the door for them to experience their emotions, giving the simple message that it is all right to grieve.

Knowing how to recognize the different stages of grief greatly assists you in providing your clients with the type of support they need. Sincerity and open communication are key to maintaining a supportive relationship with clients.

Veterinary staff members are in a position to encourage healthy coping skills in their clients. Clients look to the veterinary staff for support, assurance, understanding and validation when facing a loss. If you can assist your clients in this way, you will be laying the foundation for a natural resolution of the loss. In doing so, you will continue to maintain their respect and solidify your working relationship.

Acknowledging the Loss

In being present with clients during a loss, you help to legitimize the grief reaction and give them permission to verbalize their feelings. Many pet owners go to great lengths to appear stoic in the presence of others. In our society, death is often dealt with through denial, so it is vital that you validate the client's loss. The most beneficial thing a veterinary staff member can do for clients is to let them know that grieving for the loss of a pet is perfectly normal.

Ways of expressing condolences include sending a card, flowers or personal note to the client. What a client needs and values most from veterinary staff members is their time and presence. Being cared for and acknowledged is something a client will remember long after the flowers have wilted and the note or card has been discarded.

Veterinary staff members may feel uncomfortable in attending a grieving client. Some pet owners attribute unrealistic powers of control over life and death to their veterinarians. This is especially true for "last hope practitioners," veterinarians who are specialists in their fields. A client whose pet has cancer, and who has been referred to an internist for treatment, may have a strong need to believe that this doctor with specialized skills will be able to help the pet. This can place the veterinarian in the difficult position of conveying the limitations of treatment to the client.

Being with a client who is very tearful or angry can be an uncomfortable experience. You may worry that you will do or say the wrong thing. You may find it easier to hide behind the professional role and keep the client emotionally at a distance. This often leaves the client feeling uncared for and abandoned. A client will be less likely to return to an emotionally unsupportive veterinary facility even if miracles were performed with the deceased or terminally ill pet.

Your responsibility is not to work in the capacity of a therapist or counselor. However, your relationships with your clients can be enhanced by learning and using a variety of counseling and communication skills. By communicating effectively with your clients, you will help them to accept and resolve their losses sooner than those pet owners whose losses have not been properly acknowledged.

Useful skills and techniques that can be used to assist your clients include attending, effective listening, reflection and validation.

Attending

Without realizing it, you can make it difficult for clients to express their feelings and concerns. The way in which you sit, stand, look at or speak to them can inhibit or enhance communication.

Open posture with uncrossed arms and legs demonstrates to your clients that you are available and ready to listen. Facing them directly while maintaining comfortable eye contact sends the message that you are interested in what they have to say.

Effective Listening

Listening effectively is much more than hearing what a client is saying. Listening effectively means giving the client your complete attention and allowing space for the client to ramble, cry and show anger. You should learn to tolerate periods of silence from the client. You may feel a strong desire to fill in the silence with words. Restrain yourself. The client needs you to be there silently.

By recognizing the different components of grief, you can accept the client's expressions of anger and denial and be empathetic about the guilt and deep sadness. Whether the client's initial reaction is overt despair or quiet shock, your interactions will set the stage for the grieving process that follows.

You will find it easier to help some clients than others, and you will need to make an extra effort to support the more difficult ones. The more challenging the client, the more important it is to respond with empathy, and the more adept you will become in meeting your clients' emotional needs.

Demonstrate that you are attempting to understand what the clients are expressing by responding at appropriate intervals to their comments. Avoid using cliches or telling them that you know exactly how they feel. You don't.

Try saying, "What I hear you saying is . . . ." Let them tell you what the loss means to them. Ask the client, "How can I help you? What things have you done in the past that have supported you through a difficult time?" By asking specific questions, you will be able to identify what they need from you and enable them to begin to take care of themselves.

A Case Study

Carol was devastated after having chosen euthanasia for her ill bird and companion of 11 years. She had centered much of her life around her bird, limiting her social life and friends. Her associates and friends were sympathetic but unsupportive about her loss. In talking with her bird's veterinarian, she shared the fact that she felt a void in her life and did not know what to do.

A helpful response to such a statement would be, "You've devoted so much time and love to Pickles that it feels as though your life will be lonely and empty without him. Would it be helpful for you to consider that while a door has closed on his life, one might be opening in yours?"

This statement acknowledges the emptiness she feels, as well as the fact that she can create a new life for herself.

Reflection

When a response successfully summarizes what the client is expressing, this is called *reflection*. When you reflect clients' underlying concerns, they feel that you understand what they are saying. In addition, you can reframe the experience of loss and hopelessness into one of hope and possibility. When clients feel that hospital staff members understand the depth of the sadness, they see that others view the loss as significant.

By establishing open communication, you will be in a position to offer the kind of help that is needed. Some clients may only need to hear that they did the right thing and to be informed about burial options. Others will need emotional support and may be referred to a group or private therapist.

Validating the Loss

When your clients tell you what a loss means to them, you will need to let them know that you understand the relationship they have shared with the pet. In validating the loss, you will discover that a pet can fulfill many needs of pet owners. Be alert for key comments, such as, "We never had any children; Barney was like our child," "Ginger was my whole life," or "How will I ever feel safe alone at night without Rusty?" A pet may have served as a child to some, a best friend to others, or even as a bridge to the past. It may have accompanied the owner from college to career, to marriage, and on through other important life stages. It may have been a source of comfort during a stressful time: a divorce, loss of a loved one, a move, or a change in jobs.

The current loss can trigger the remembrance of past losses. This compound effect may overwhelm the client. Clients often report being surprised by the memory of past losses. The more closely connected the pet was to the past loss, the more difficult it can be for the client.

3 Case Studies

A woman who lost her baby to Sudden Infant Death Syndrome acquired a puppy to help her through the loss. The puppy was something to cuddle and need her. Though it was by no means a replacement for the child she had lost, it helped her through the experience. When her dog died, she not only grieved for the loss of him, but for the loss of her child as well.

Another client who lost a dog that had been her constant companion remarked that his death was more difficult for her than the recent loss of her mother, with whom she had been close.

A Vietnam veteran who had chosen euthanasia for his 17-year-old, very ill cat shared that the cat was the first living thing he was able to learn to love again after returning home from the war.

Validation of the loss occurs when you accurately summarize what the loss means to the client, based on the client's own statements. By considering the examples below, you can begin to form an idea of what you need to say to your clients.

"Losing your dog reminds you of the loss of your child. It must be a very painful time for you."

"Your dog was a significant member of your family. The unconditional love you received is a gift that people are not always able to give one another."

"It is difficult for me to imagine what Vietnam was like, but I do know that this cat was very special to you. She has given you a gift that no one else could give you."

You will use your own words to convey messages of understanding and empathy toward your clients. The idea is to listen and express back to the client the core significance of the loss. Validating a client's loss helps to make the client feel special and cared for by the veterinarian and the hospital staff.

Achieving Closure

The perfect way to end a conversation with a grieving client is to give a directive. For example, "I would like you to go home, get some rest and then think about the options we discussed." Accompanying the directive with a caring statement reassures clients that you empathize and that their feelings are important.

Many clients take comfort in thinking about ways in which to honor their pets. For example, clients can donate to a specific cause in honor of a pet, plant a rose bush near the burial site, or create a scrapbook of memories shared with the pet.

The following suggestions may be helpful in assisting your clients.

- *Provide facial tissues* (Kleenex) in any room where a bereaved pet owner may need them.

- *Schedule appointment times to allow for additional time to be spent with a bereaved pet owner* or one whose pet is seriously ill.

- *Create a brochure that includes all available support information* (pet loss support groups, private therapists, hotlines, burial information, literature on pet loss, etc). Make the brochure available to clients anticipating a loss as well as those experiencing one.

- *Send a card or flowers immediately after the loss.* Late arrivals can be painful reminders for clients.

- *Collect any fees owed before the euthanasia procedure is performed.* A client will find it awkward to have to regain composure and pay a bill after the emotional experience of saying goodbye to a beloved pet.

- *Let your clients know that you and the rest of the staff are available to assist them,* before and after loss of a pet.

Most pet owners have questions regarding their pets' illness and need reassurance that they did the right thing.

- If possible, *maintain a private area in which clients can say goodbye to their pet, grieve or regain composure.* If such an area is not available, consider allowing extra time in the examination room before a loss and afterward.

- When attending to the patient, *make certain that the owner can tell that the pet is comfortable and cared for.* A simple gesture, such as placing a towel on a cold examination table, can demonstrate your compassion for the patient. If you send a final bill to the client, be sure it does not arrive on the same day as the card or flowers.

Effects of Patient Loss
on Veterinary Staff

As difficult as the loss of a pet may be for a client, the loss of a patient may be difficult for the staff and veterinarian as well. Pets generally live one-fifth of the lifespan of people. Because euthanasia is an acceptable and legal means of terminating an animal's life, veterinary practitioners and their staff face a stress that is unknown to most other medical practitioners.

Each member of the staff has a personal set of beliefs and feelings regarding the issue of loss. Some may feel awkward attending a grieving client. Others may have unresolved feelings about pets they have lost themselves. Most people in the veterinary field have a love for animals and want to help them. Few consider the effect of the loss of a patient upon themselves.

When assisting bereaved pet owners, staff members may feel emotions similar to those the client experiences. Learn how to empathize and assist in a caring manner while still maintaining emotional distance. The following steps will help you in this process.

- *Take a team approach to cases in which euthanasia is an option.* This can alleviate some of the feelings of failure and grief regarding loss of a patient.

- *Create and participate in a support group for veterinary staff.* This is a forum for airing private feelings and receiving feedback from peers.

- *Refer pet owners to a pet loss support group.* This provides clients with a safe place to share feelings and validates the fact that the loss of a patient is a real and important consideration for everyone involved.

- *Encourage open communication among staff members,* confrontation of personal feelings and beliefs surrounding death, as well as self-examination regarding the emotional reaction to the loss of a patient. This helps to eliminate guilt and other bad feelings.

Veterinary staff members have the opportunity to present the best their practice has to offer when a client is facing the crisis of losing a treasured pet. You can play a significant role in assisting the client through an emotionally difficult time, thereby solidifying your working relationship with the pet owner. Clients who respect the veterinarian and staff will speak highly of them to others, refer other pet owners to the practice and return with new pets.

The loss of a pet is stressful for the entire staff, as well as the pet owner. By confronting their feelings, staff members can work through their emotions and maintain a healthy perspective on the roles they play within the practice. Pet loss is an opportunity for everyone concerned to grow emotionally and to solidify working relationships.

Children and Pet Loss

Our society tends to remove children from experiences of death and dying. In past generations, death was viewed as part of life and was present in the home environment because grandparents often died at home among family and friends. Nowadays, relatives usually die in hospitals and nursing homes, places where children rarely go. Because a pet's lifespan is about one-fifth of a person's, it is realistic to expect that a child will witness the dying process of a family pet.

Parents may seek your advice on how to explain the loss to their child. They may ask you for options available within your office setting for saying goodbye to their pet. Sometimes a parent will need a referral to a therapist or support group that can assist the child in adjusting to the loss.

What should children be told? Because a child's interpretation of death varies considerably with the child's age, a thorough understanding of how death is experienced by children of various ages is important. Even very young children can sense when something is wrong and will benefit from explanations in understandable terms. It is healthy for children to grieve openly and to express their feelings about loss. This should be encouraged.

When the loss of a pet is a child's first experience with death, concerns about mortality, fear and abandonment arise. Open, honest communication helps a child to build a secure foundation for facing future losses.

Pet Loss: A Family Issue

When a pet is dying, sending a child away to be with friends or relatives can be traumatic, especially if the child and the pet shared a bond. The child's feelings of abandonment may be intensified. Children need to be part of the family in painful times, as well as in the best of times. Sharing feelings with parents and siblings validates the right to have those feelings and teaches children that grief does not have to be hidden or endured alone.

Grief should not be viewed as shameful. Sharing tears as well as laughter is healthy and normal. Children learn that it is good to express such emotions when they witness open grieving by someone they love and respect. This gives them permission to face their own feelings when the time comes.

Shared grief can be a catalyst in promoting a healthy family unit. Support groups and counselors who specialize in grief and loss can assist a family in coming to terms with such issues. Adults who show respect for children's feelings help them to develop confidence and self-esteem.

The Importance of Truth

Though it is tempting to avoid discussing the issue surrounding death, this is not in children's best interests. Lying about the fate of a pet may be well-intentioned but is unfair because it excludes children from the decision-making process, takes away their right to say goodbye and ignores their need to do so. As children mature and have questions about the loss, they may discover the lie and feel angry or betrayed by those individuals whom they trusted the most.

Children need a safe, secure environment in which to ask questions, receive answers and express feelings of anger, sorrow, guilt and fear about death. As painful as it may be for an adult to see a child grieving, the child should be allowed to work through the grief. When a pet dies, the circumstances should be explained honestly. Of course, unpleasant details can be left out. Best are clear, direct answers stated in a way that the child can understand.

Openness and honesty encourage the child to ask questions. Sometimes a child will ask questions immediately, but it is not uncommon for a child to ask them over the course of a year or more. Reminders such as a dead animal on the road may trigger more thoughts and questions about the loss of a pet. As children mature, their knowledge expands. They need to integrate what they learn about death with the rest of their knowledge about the world. They do this best when they feel free to ask questions and know they will receive straightforward answers.

Individual Responses to Pet Loss

Children's reactions to losing a pet vary according to their age, as well as their relationship with the animal. Very young children often view their pets as playmates, imagining that they can talk and play games. Pets may take the place of a brother or a sister for children without siblings. Children may think of their pet as a best friend, someone to confide in, someone who loves them.

Children may distance themselves from their pets, much as they do from other family members at a time when they are trying to establish autonomy and develop their own identity. Peers may become more important in their lives. This does not mean that they no longer care for their pet; they may still share a deep kinship with it. Parents should ask children what the loss means to them and should not assume that children do not care because they have been less actively involved than they were in the past.

Cognitive Age and the Effects of Loss

Children are affected by loss according to their level of cognitive development. Children as young as 2 years old can experience feelings of grief and sorrow. At this age, their feelings are often related to ones of abandonment and they particularly need help to feel safe and secure during a loss.

When children reach preschool age, their understanding of loss is linked with imaginary play. They may believe that when a pet dies, it is only asleep. These children need help in understanding the finality of death and that the pet will not wake up or return home.

When children reach elementary school age, they are able to conceive of death as the final stage of life. However, they may think it cannot happen to them. These children may think that a pet died because it was bad. They may blame themselves for the death, believing that a pet died or ran away because of something they did, did not do, or wished for in a fit of anger. Reassuring children that feelings of anger are normal and will not cause a pet's disappearance or demise will help them cope with the loss.

As children mature, they realize that death is a part of life's cycle and that every living thing dies. They should be reminded that the majority of people live for a long time, and that, in the unlikely event that something happened to their parents, they would be cared for by someone else.

A preteen child searches for the meaning of life and ways of coping with loss. A child at this stage of development needs open communication and encouragement to share feelings of pain.

Extreme Responses to Loss

If the grieving process is compounded by other problems, a child may consider suicide. A child who even hints at this possibility must be taken seriously. Immediate intervention is needed. The child should be taken to a therapist or crisis center to validate the pain and be taught to cope with it.

Recognizing Hidden Grief

A child's feelings about the loss of a pet may not always be obvious to an adult. The child may display anger at situations and objects not directly related to the loss. Children who are usually well behaved may display aggression at home or in school as they try to cope with their grief. Children who feel abandoned may express anger at the pet, saying "I never liked him anyway," though they are really hurting inside.

Because children tend to show little immediate grief, they may seem to be unaffected by the loss of a pet. They may question intensively for a period, and then not mention the subject for a while. As painful as it may be for other family members to have the subject brought up again and again, children need patience and understanding while working through the process of grieving.

Adults may underplay the significance of the pet's death in an effort to minimize the child's pain. If adults treat the death or loss of a pet as unimportant, children may fear that no one would care if they too were to die.

The following example shows how a family dealt with a child's unhappiness and fear resulting from euthanasia of her pet.

A Case Study

According to her mother, 9-year-old Emily's best friend was her cat, Harvey. Harvey disappeared one day, and was discovered hiding under the front porch of their house. He was injured. The veterinarian who examined Harvey gave a very poor prognosis for recovery. Treatment would be extensive and costly. The family discussed their options and included Emily in the discussion. Emily's mother said that she could not afford the costly treatment and was concerned that, even if she could, they would put Harvey through more misery with little hope for recovery. The family opted for euthanasia. Emily was permitted to say her final goodbyes to Harvey.

A few weeks after Harvey's death Emily continued to cry intermittently. She had difficulty concentrating in school and remained at home instead of playing with her friends. Emily's mother sought the help of a counselor.

Emily told the counselor that this was the first time someone she loved had died. She said it hurt inside and she was afraid it would not stop. The counselor asked her if she remembered how much it hurt inside the day Harvey died. She said it hurt a lot, more than it did right now. The counselor told Emily that as the days went by she would still continue to miss Harvey, but she would feel better every day, and soon she would be able to remember him without feeling sad.

Finally, Emily told the counselor that she was afraid that if she became ill, her mother would be unable to afford to take care of her. When this fact was brought to her mother's attention, she assured Emily that her first priority was Emily and that she would always provide for her. She also reminded Emily that Harvey's treatment would have been extensive and painful and his chances for full recovery were not good.

Emily was able to accept this information and soon resumed her normal activities. She and her mother found ways to memorialize Harvey. Emily named a favorite stuffed animal after him, and she and her mother held a ceremony for Harvey.

Emily did very well working through her first loss. Her success can be attributed to a supportive family who took time to include her in important decisions, encouraged her to express her feelings, and got help for her when she was having difficulties. As a result, Emily developed coping skills that she will be able to use throughout her life.

Choosing the Right Words

In working with children, correct terminology is particularly important. For example, saying that a pet has been "put to sleep" instead of using the medical term "euthanized" is confusing for a child, who may be afraid of burying a "sleeping" pet. The child may resist falling asleep for fear of not waking up again.

Euthanasia should be explained to children in terms they can comprehend. A child could be told that the pet will be put to death with an injection of a powerful medication given

by the veterinarian. Stress that this injection is only available to animals and is not the same type of injection a child
receives at the pediatrician's office.

Helping Through Sharing

If a pet is to be euthanized, the veterinarian and parents
should offer the child the options of saying goodbye to the
pet beforehand, viewing the pet's body afterward, or being
present for the procedure. Children who are prepared in
advance and who can understand the procedure should be
allowed to attend if they so desire. They should be given
support during the procedure.

Children's attitudes about pets and their reactions to loss
vary with age. Understanding a child's process of development allows parents and other caregivers to help a child
through the process of grieving. Avoiding the issue, telling
lies or trivializing the loss could have a devastating effect,
and does not teach the child about how to cope with grief.
By helping the child to deal with issues of separation and
loss, parents and professionals can provide a solid foundation for dealing with the life cycle, which is a process of
endings and new beginnings.

Pet Loss and
the Elderly

In today's society, a pet is often the sole companion for an
elderly person. Many elderly people have lost their spouses,
and their immediate family may live far from them. A pet
can enrich an older person's life by providing companion-
ship, affection and a sense of being needed.

When older persons move to a retirement home, the pet
may not be allowed to accompany them. Elderly pets are not
easily adoptable, and often owners request euthanasia

rather than relinquish the pet to a shelter. This may present a moral dilemma for the office staff. Owners may experience a deep sense of inadequacy and loss of self-esteem when faced with giving up a pet and having the unpleasant choices of placing it in another home or euthanizing it if no home can be found. Long-term clients may turn to the veterinarian for assistance when facing such a choice.

If pets are allowed at the retirement home, owners may not be able to get another after the original pet dies. Then not only do elderly persons grieve the loss of a cherished pet, they must also adjust to never being able to care for a pet again.

A Link with the Past

A pet can represent a link with the past, especially for the elderly person. Often the responsibilities of pet care were shared with a spouse who is now deceased. The loss of the pet can trigger intense memories of the previous loss and open wounds that go beyond the attachment to the animal.

A Case Study

Mrs. Potts and her husband of 30 years shared the care of a poodle for the last 7 years of Mr. Potts' life. His wish was to have the dog's ashes and his ashes scattered together when they both died. At his death, Mrs. Potts promised her husband that she would provide loving care for the pet for the rest of its life. The dog continued to live for another 7 years. With time his hearing and eyesight failed and he lost bladder control. Mrs. Potts found it increasingly difficult to care for the dog, especially because she was experiencing age-related problems herself. The veterinarian recommended that she consider euthanasia. Recalling the promise that she had made to her husband, she was reluctant to do so.

Finally, with support from the veterinary staff, Mrs. Potts was able to make the decision that was right for both her and her pet. If the office staff had been less supportive and understanding, Mrs. Potts might have experienced more confusion and guilt in making the choice for euthanasia.

Loneliness of Aging

As a person ages, his or her support system suffers. Friends and family may be gone or ill and emotionally unavailable. A diminishing support system can intensify feelings of despair, loneliness and isolation. The elderly person who has lost a pet may become depressed.

An elderly person's entire day may be centered around care of the pet. Feeding, walking and playing with the pet provide activity and exercise for the owner. In addition, the pet may be a source of security in the home, scaring away intruders or attracting the owner's attention in the event of a fire. For older people living alone, isolated from human interaction, a pet can be a source of tactile warmth and unconditional affection. When the pet dies, daily routines are altered and simple pleasures of daily living can be seriously diminished.

Responding to Special Needs of the Elderly

Simply getting to the veterinary office may pose a problem for elderly clients. They may be forced to rely on cab service, which can be costly, especially for clients on a fixed income. Your office may consider offering these clients home visits for routine injections or medication administration.

When an elderly client has not come in for the pet's yearly examination and vaccinations, consider a telephone call to check on your patient and, at this time, to offer the client options for continued care. You might say, "We've noticed that Skippy didn't come in for his annual visit and wondered if you were having difficulties with transportation. If so, we sometimes arrange for the doctor to make a house call. Please let us know if you are interested." You may feel more comfortable sending the client a reminder note including this information.

In addition to transportation needs, try to assess your elderly clients for vision and hearing impairments. Home care instructions may have to be written in large type and examination results explained carefully, slowly and loudly. Ask the client to repeat the information back to ensure complete understanding.

Ordinary doors, walkways, and parking lots may be difficult for the elderly client to negotiate, especially when leading a pet or carrying it in a bulky carrier. Assisting these persons in restraining a pet, opening office and car doors, and carrying pet food and supplies says that you value their business and care for them as individuals.

When an elderly client is faced with loss of a pet, certain factors complicate the response to the loss and have implications for your office staff. The current loss almost always awakens memories of past losses, compounding feelings of sorrow and loneliness. Housing restrictions, the client's age and health, as well as financial considerations pose obstacles to pet replacement. In the aged, loss of a constant companion and best friend can have devastating effects from which it may be difficult to recover.

Assess these clients carefully for their ability to come to your office, understand instructions and read medication labels or information pamphlets. Extend yourself to elderly clients by offering physical assistance to and from car to office or by arranging in-home visits when necessary. Offer senior discounts for services if possible.

Small kindnesses go a long way toward making a client feel worthwhile and cared for. For a client whose self-esteem may already be compromised by a dwindling support system and personal health problems, a show of concern and respect is always appreciated.

Extreme Responses to Loss of a Pet

Infrequently the loss of a pet triggers an unusual or abnormal response in certain clients. You may see some of these behaviors acted out in your office or you may recognize trouble in the verbal context of a client's telephone message. Grief responses carried to the extreme become abnormal and may pose problems for the staff-client relationship. If left unchecked, they can progress to serious problems for the client, their family and significant others. Following are some "red flag" situations to alert you to the need for additional interventions on behalf of your client.

Anger

Anger is a common response seen in clients who have lost or are anticipating the loss of a pet. In most cases, anger is short-lived and dissipates once they have had time to assimilate all the facts related to the pet's illness or death.

When the anger is projected outward, it may remain there in a holding pattern that actually protects a person from the impact of their own rage. If a client were guilty of unintentional neglect contributing to the pet's demise, when that knowledge breaks through the defenses, they may finally turn the anger upon themselves. Some clients may not have people with whom to discuss their feelings and may be completely unaware that others also have experienced feelings of anger and shame under similar circumstances. These individuals may experience such intense feelings of self-loathing and loneliness that they entertain thoughts of suicide. A suicide gesture is a real possibility when unchecked anger progresses to rage, and the rage (previously directed toward someone else) is now turned upon themselves.

Prolonged Despair

Persistent despair (loss of all hope that things will ever be good again) is not part of the normal grieving process. It may require the professional intervention of a skilled therapist. Clients who have a weak or absent support system may regard their pet as the only one who cares if they live or die. Once the pet is gone, these clients may feel such intense loneliness that their will to participate in normal daily activities is seriously undermined. In addition, guilt associated with the death of the pet can damage self-esteem so that they may disengage from social commitments, break off personal relationships, and even jeopardize their livelihood by failing to report to work.

Guilt

Guilt is experienced by most pet owners who decide to euthanize their pets. Even in cases where the pet was loved and well cared for and euthanasia was chosen to prevent undue pain and suffering, doubt may remain in the client's mind about the timing of the euthanasia. A client may say, "I know Sugar might have enjoyed another week or two of life if I hadn't jumped in and played God . . . maybe even a month or two!" Similarly, the client may imagine that euthanasia was delayed for too long: "It was so selfish of me to hang on! I think Mugsy suffered needlessly because I was too selfish to let him go at the right time."

Clients who cannot afford treatment must deal with the guilt and feelings of inadequacy related to financial constraints. These clients must be told that they have done all within their means to provide the best care and treatment for their pet and that you understand their need to discontinue treatment. You must validate the deep sadness they are experiencing. Try saying, "I realize this is a very tough decision for you. If additional testing and treatment would compromise the welfare of the rest of your family, you should not pursue it. I know how much you love Suzy and what she means to your family. Your love for Suzy will not be diminished if you are unable to extend yourself financially now."

A Case Study

Six months before coming to the veterinary office, Pam noticed a small lump in Petey's neck. She was frightened, but denied to herself that anything could be seriously wrong. The lump is larger now and is found to be an inoperable carcinoma.

Pam is very angry and hostile, accusing the doctor of missing the lump on the last examination. She refuses to pay her bill and is considering a lawsuit for negligence. You tell her about a local pet loss support group, but she decides not to attend.

Pam is feeling guilty about her failure to seek treatment when she first noticed the lump 6 months ago. She finds it easier to displace the anger and blame the veterinary office rather than accept her share of responsibility. Contacting Pam by telephone would probably be counterproductive, but consider writing a letter acknowledging her pending loss and sadness. You might say, "I know how much you love Petey and what good care you've given him over the years. This is a very difficult time for you, and if you would like the doctor to see Petey again, or if you'd like referral for consultation, please let us know."

Acknowledging Pam's love for Petey and the good care she has given him in the past might assuage some of her guilt over the present situation. By expressing your concern for Pam, even in the face of her anger and threats, you leave the door open for her to bring Petey back to your office for the duration of his illness.

After a week, Pam calls your office for an appointment. When she comes in, she is calm, attentive and reasonable. She is now able to assimilate the information and recommendations offered and make plans for Petey's immediate care. A referral to the pet loss support group is appropriate, and she will probably attend. You might add, "If you don't feel comfortable in groups, I can give you the names of individuals who might be of some help to you. It's your choice, but understand that you don't need to go through this alone."

Problems Associated with Missing Pets

Clients whose pets are missing are at risk for experiencing any of these extreme responses. There is often anger and rage at the unknown person who may have abducted the pet or found it and failed to search for its owner or turn it over to an agency that would do so. The client may experience intense guilt over having left the pet unattended, left a gate or door open, or any act of neglect that resulted in the pet's disappearance.

These individuals have difficulty obtaining closure on the event because days and weeks may pass without any information on the welfare and whereabouts of the pet. With time, guilt intensifies rather than dissipates the way it does in the normal grieving process. Clients may discuss their feelings about the missing pet or may withhold the information because they are ashamed about what has happened.

The client may appear overly concerned and protective of the remaining pets, even during routine examinations and procedures. These clients could benefit from a pet loss support group, where they can share feelings of shame, guilt and sorrow with others who have experienced pet loss under a variety of circumstances. They need help to gain closure on the loss; this type of loss does not heal readily with time alone.

Clients whose pets who are victims of accidents, such as vehicular trauma or poisoning, may have prolonged grief. For these individuals, guilt feelings can be intense and pervasive, continuing for weeks and months without abatement. Be sensitive to the special needs of these clients, who are often unable to move from the guilt phase of their grief without the assistance of a mental health professional.

A Case Study

A woman of comfortable means brought her toy poodle, Pierre, home from the groomer. While she was transferring grocery bags from her car to the kitchen, Pierre barked once and disappeared behind the house. Pierre was obedient to heel and had never left his mistress' side before. This time he had not only left the property but he disappeared without a trace.

Pierre's owner searched everywhere for him. She took out advertisements, went from door to door and drove endless miles calling for him. As time went by, she became more obsessed with Pierre's disappearance, and her frantic and desperate search cost her many hundreds of dollars and eventually her marriage. Her intense feelings of guilt were persistent and unassuagable.

Finally she engaged the services of a psychic for missing children who was able to construct in some detail the events leading to the disappearance and demise of Pierre. With the psychic's assistance, she was able to lay her guilt and self-blame to rest and attain some closure. Extreme measures were required to finalize the loss for this client. Most clients can achieve significant closure in the healing environment of a pet loss support group.

Clients Who Abuse Alcohol

There may be clients in your practice whom you suspect of being under the influence of alcohol or another substance. An odor of alcohol on the breath, an unsteady gait and slurred speech are the hallmarks of alcohol intoxication. A "tipsy" client making a routine visit to your office may pose no problem for office staff. However, this same client may present difficulties during a real or perceived emergency. The client may overreact to statements about diagnosis, prognosis and recommended treatment, and may display emotional extremes, such as hysteria, while demanding that you make unreasonable or unrealistic interventions on behalf of the pet. This client will have difficulty making decisions and, unless absolutely necessary, should not be pressed to do so.

Keep explanations brief and instructions simple. Attempt to secure a ride home for them by saying, "You look unsteady on your feet. I'm wondering if I might telephone a cab or a friend to take you home." Make a notation of your offer in the record in case your judgment is called into question at a later date. In any case, contact the client the next day to discuss the examination results in detail and to give additional instructions for the care of the pet. Decisions regarding euthanasia or extensive treatment might be discussed at this time if the client seems focused and attentive during the conversation.

Because alcohol is relatively inexpensive and readily available, people may be tempted to take a drink to soften the edges of reality during stressful periods in life. In fact, alcohol is a depressant and therefore is a poor choice for fending off feelings of fear and loneliness. Drinking may initially produce a short-lived feeling of euphoria. Drinking to excess more often results in dysphoria (disquiet, restlessness, malaise) accompanied by reality distortions and impaired judgment. Alcohol also interferes with sleep patterns. The loss of sleep can further reduce the ability to cope with the emotional roller coaster that embodies the grief process.

Compounded Loss

When faced with loss of a pet, the owner is often reminded (while awake or in dreams) of losses from the past, both human and animal. This compounded effect of past and present loss can feel so overpowering that a client may respond in a way that seems quite out of proportion to the current facts. When this occurs, you might say, "I can see that you are really troubled and worried about Tinker. Have you had any previous experiences with loss in your life?"

Sometimes an invitation to talk about a previous pet loss elicits information regarding past loss of family and friends, the demise of a relationship or loss of a job. If the information is forthcoming, you can tell the client, "I know that when faced with the loss of a pet that you love, you can be reminded of other painful losses you've experienced, and this can hurt more than if you were dealing with a single loss. Don't be surprised if you are suddenly recalling sad times from the past. Just know that it is very natural, at a time like this, to remember family and friends who are no longer with you. Try talking things over with a close friend, or, if you'd like, I can give you some referrals for counseling that might help you get through this difficult time."

Recognizing and Responding to Signals

A client may convey feelings of deep despair either verbally or through body language. Such statements as, "Maggie is the only friend I have in the world. I don't know how I can face another day without her by my side," or "Nothing matters now that Barney is dying. It will kill me to bring him in for euthanasia. I might as well be dead too" should alert you to the need for outside professional evaluation and treatment.

You must determine if these clients have a reliable, concerned friend or relative who can stay with them, particularly if you have doubts about their safety if left alone. Make appropriate referrals and offer to call for an appointment before they leave the office. Do this openly to encourage trust and open communication. Sometimes just knowing that an appointment has been arranged has a calming and reassuring effect. Make every effort to secure the first appointment available and, if possible, telephone the client the next day for a "welfare check" and reminder of the appointment date and time. Extract a promise from the client that they will contact the crisis intervention hotline if they experience overwhelming loneliness and sadness. Make certain they leave with the hotline telephone number in an accessible place.

If the client refuses any referrals or assistance and you sense that he is a danger to himself, you may need to resort to police escort of this client to a local psychiatric clinic for evaluation and treatment. This may seem to be an extreme measure, but it could save a life. You might say to the client, "I know that you do not want to accept a referral for help, but I am so concerned about you that I will notify the police for assistance in getting you the help you need. I really do care about you and don't want anything bad to happen to you." Remember that extreme actions sometimes call for extreme reactions to prevent future pain and suffering.

Referring to Mental
Health Professionals:
When and Why

Clients experiencing intense anger, despair and guilt often benefit from professional intervention outside of your office. Maintain a list of counselors and support groups for referral of clients experiencing grief associated with pet loss. Your local mental health department can assist you. They can also provide you with information regarding community-based agencies and resources available on a low-fee or no-fee basis. The Delta Society in Renton, Washington, maintains a list of pet loss support counselors and groups throughout the country. Assembling a community referral file for your clients may take some time and effort, but this special service conveys the hospital staff's concern for their safety and well-being.

Conclusion

While you may never encounter a client in a full-blown psychotic episode, you should be familiar with the circumstances related to pet loss that can jeopardize your clients' well-being. One client may handle loss of a pet with ease, while another may experience a crisis so overwhelming as to be life threatening.

Clients are individuals with widely divergent personal histories and coping skills. While the greatest percentage of your time and effort is, of course, devoted to your patients, take time to notice the emotional status of your clients. A little caring can go a long way toward guiding a client through the grieving process. You will feel good about making a positive connection with your clients and will gain a reputation for the veterinary office as one that is responsive and sensitive to the needs of both patients and clients.

Recommended Reading

Brackenridge SS and Elkins AD: Euthanasia and patient death. *Vet Pract Staff* 4(4):1,8-10, 1992.

Diagnostic and Statistical Manual of Mental Disorders. 3rd ed. Am Psychiat Assn, Cambridge, MA, 1987.

Grollman EA: *Talking About Death.* 3rd ed. Beacon Press, Boston, 1990.

Guntzelman J and Rieger M: Helping pet owners with the euthanasia decision. *Vet Med* 88:26-34, 1993.

Guntzelman J and Rieger M: Supporting clients who are grieving the death of a pet. *Vet Med* 88:35-41, 1993.

Hart LA and Hart BL: Grief and stress from so many animal deaths. *Compan Anim Pract* 1:20-21, 1987.

Kay WJ *et al: Euthanasia of the Companion Animal.* Charles Press, Philadelphia, 1988.

Kubler-Ross E: *On Death and Dying.* Collier Books, New York, 1969.

Ross CB: Pet loss and the human/companion animal bond. Master's thesis, Sonoma State Univ, 1987.

Notes

Notes

Index

A

anger, grieving process, 141, 166
appointments, scheduling, 29-35
audiovisuals, client education, 135

B

bargaining, grieving process, 141
biologics, 81

C

castration, time of, 8
children and pet loss, 155-162
client education, 131-138
  audiovisuals, 135
  books, 136
  handouts and brochures, 133, 134
  microscopic viewing, 136
client relations, 111-117
  communicating with clients, 112, 132
  interacting with clients, 114-116
client visits, scheduling, 29-35
computers, use in practice, 107-110
controlled substances, 62
costs, drugs and supplies, 75-81

D

denial, grieving process, 140
dental care, 5
dismissing an employee, 104
dress code, 97

E

ear care, 5
economic order quantity, 76-80
economics of ordering supplies, 75-81
elderly and pet loss, 162-166
emergencies, 23-28
employee supervision, 87-105
  dismissals, 104
  dress code, 97
  firing, 104
  fringe benefits, 98
  handling personnel problems, 101
  hiring, 90-97
  interviewing, 95-97
  job descriptions, 97, 98
  performance reviews, 102
  personal leave, 98
  scheduling work hours, 99-101
  stress management, 103, 104
  time cards, 98
  training new employees, 97-99
euthanasia consent forms, 49-51
eye care, 6